Advanced Imaging in Ischemic and Hemorrhagic Stroke

Editors

JOSEPH J. GEMMETE
ZACHARY M. WILSECK

NEUROIMAGING CLINICS OF NORTH AMERICA

www.neuroimaging.theclinics.com

Consulting Editor
SURESH K. MUKHERJI

May 2024 • Volume 34 • Number 2

ELSEVIER

1600 John F. Kennedy Boulevard • Suite 1800 • Philadelphia, Pennsylvania, 19103-2899

http://www.neuroimaging.theclinics.com

NEUROIMAGING CLINICS OF NORTH AMERICA Volume 34, Number 2
May 2024 ISSN 1052-5149, ISBN 13: 978-0-443-13133-2

Editor: John Vassallo (j.vassallo@elsevier.com)
Developmental Editor: Saswoti Nath

Neuroimaging Clinics of North America (ISSN 1052-5149) is published quarterly by Elsevier Inc., 360 Park Avenue South, New York, NY 10010-1710. Months of issue are February, May, August, and November. Business and editorial offices: 1600 John F. Kennedy Blvd., Suite 1800, Philadelphia, PA 19103-2899. Business and editorial offices: 6277 Sea Harbor Drive, Orlando, FL 32887-4800. Periodicals postage paid at New York, NY, and additional mailing offices. Subscription prices are USD 430 per year for US individuals, USD 100 per year for US students and residents, USD 493 per year for Canadian individuals, USD 573 per year for international individuals, USD 100 per year for Canadian students and residents and USD 260 per year for foreign students and residents. For institutional access pricing please contact Customer Service via the contact information below. To receive student/resident rate, orders must be accompanied by name of affiliated institution, date of term, and the *signature* of program/residency coordinator on institution letterhead. Orders will be billed at individual rate until proof of status is received. Foreign air speed delivery is included in all *Clinics* subscription prices. All prices are subject to change without notice. POSTMASTER: Send address changes to *Neuroimaging Clinics of North America*, Elsevier Health Sciences Division, Subscription **Customer Service, 3251 Riverport Lane, Maryland Heights, MO 63043. Telephone: 1-800-654-2452 (U.S. and Canada); 314-447-8871 (outside U.S. and Canada). Fax: 314-447-8029. E-mail: journalscustomer-service-usa@elsevier.com (for print support); journalsonlinesupport-usa@elsevier.com (for online support)**.

Reprints. For copies of 100 or more of articles in this publication, please contact the Commercial Reprints Department, Elsevier Inc., 360 Park Avenue South, New York, NY 10010-1710. Tel.: 212-633-3874; Fax: 212-633-3820; E-mail: reprints@elsevier.com.

Neuroimaging Clinics of North America is covered by *Excerpta Medical/EMBASE,* the RSNA Index of Imaging Literature, *MEDLINE/PubMed (Index Medicus),* MEDLINE/MEDLARS, SciSearch, Research Alert, and Neuroscience Citation Index.

PROGRAM OBJECTIVE

The goal of *Neuroimaging Clinics of North America* is to keep practicing radiologists and radiology residents up to date with current clinical practice in radiology by providing timely articles reviewing the state of the art in patient care.

TARGET AUDIENCE

Practicing radiologists, radiology residents, and other healthcare professionals who utilize neuroimaging findings to provide patient care.

LEARNING OBJECTIVES

1. Review the vital and time-sensitive role of magnetic resonance imaging (MRI)-based biomarkers in understanding and managing hemorrhagic strokes.
2. Discuss the clinical care for acute ischemic stroke and its evolution.
3. Recognize the variety of modern intraoperative imaging modalities available for cerebrovascular surgery.

ACCREDITATION

The Elsevier Office of Continuing Medical Education (EOCME) is accredited by the Accreditation Council for Continuing Medical Education (ACCME) to provide continuing medical education for physicians.

The EOCME designates this journal-based CME activity for a maximum of 10 *AMA PRA Category 1 Credit*(s)™. Physicians should claim only the credit commensurate with the extent of their participation in the activity.

All other healthcare professionals requesting continuing education credit for this enduring material will be issued a certificate of participation.

DISCLOSURE OF CONFLICTS OF INTEREST

The EOCME assesses conflict of interest with its instructors, faculty, planners, and other individuals who are in a position to control the content of CME activities. All relevant conflicts of interest that are identified are thoroughly vetted by EOCME for fair balance, scientific objectivity, and patient care recommendations. EOCME is committed to providing its learners with CME activities that promote improvements or quality in healthcare and not a specific proprietary business or a commercial interest.

The planning committee, staff, authors, and editors listed below have identified no financial relationships or relationships to products or devices they or their spouse/life partner have with commercial interest related to the content of this CME activity:

Ramez N. Abdalla, MD, PhD; Mohamad M. Alzein; Sameer A. Ansari, MD, PhD; Momodou G. Bah, MPH; Donald R. Cantrell, MD, PhD; Neeraj Chaudhary, MD; Huanwen Chen, MD; Thomas L. Chenevert, PhD; Ephraim Church, MD; Marco Colasurdo, MD; Ehsan Dolwati, MD; Max Fleigner; Chanju Fritch, MD; Joseph J. Gemmete, MD; Andres Gudino-Vega, MD; Katherine Guijarro-Falcon, MD; Richard Keep, PhD; Sravanthi Koduri, MD; Kothainayaki Kulanthaivelu; Leanne Y. Lin, MD, MPHS; Michelle Littlejohn; Jacob M. Miller, BSE; Luis E. Noboa; Aditya Pandey, MD; Sreehari Panicker, MS; Abhinav Patel, MD; Venkatakrishna Rajajee, MBBS; Saurabh Rohatgi, MD; Edgar A. Samaniego, MD, MS; Sebastian Sanchez, MD; Pamela W. Schaefer, MD; Ali Shaibani, MD; Anil Vasireddi, MD; D. Andrew Wilkinson, MD, MS; Zachary M. Wilseck, MD; Guohua Xi, MD

The planning committee, staff, authors, and editors listed below have identified financial relationships or relationships to products or devices they or their spouse/life partner have with commercial interest related to the content of this CME activity:

Dheeraj Gandhi, MBBS, MD: *Research Support*: MicroVention Inc., NoNO Inc.

UNAPPROVED/OFF-LABEL USE DISCLOSURE

The EOCME requires CME faculty to disclose to the participants:
1. When products or procedures being discussed are off-label, unlabelled, experimental, and/or investigational (not US Food and Drug Administration [FDA] approved); and
2. Any limitations on the information presented, such as data that are preliminary or that represent ongoing research, interim analyses, and/or unsupported opinions. Faculty may discuss information about pharmaceutical agents that is outside of FDA-approved labelling. This information is intended solely for CME and is not intended to promote off-label use of these medications. If you have any questions, contact the medical affairs department of the manufacturer for the most recent prescribing information.

TO ENROLL

To enroll in the *Neuroimaging Clinics of North America* Continuing Medical Education program, call customer service at 1-800-654-2452 or sign up online at http://www.theclinics.com/home/cme. The CME program is available to subscribers for an additional annual fee of USD 254.00.

METHOD OF PARTICIPATION

In order to claim credit, participants must complete the following:

1. Complete enrolment as indicated above.
2. Read the activity.
3. Complete the CME Test and Evaluation. Participants must achieve a score of 70% on the test. All CME Tests and Evaluations must be completed online.

CME INQUIRIES/SPECIAL NEEDS
For all CME inquiries or special needs, please contact elsevierCME@elsevier.com.

NEUROIMAGING CLINICS OF NORTH AMERICA

SERIES OF RELATED INTEREST

Advances in Clinical Radiology
Available at: https://www.advancesinclinicalradiology.com/
MRI Clinics of North America
Available at: https://www.mri.theclinics.com/
Neuroimaging Clinics
Available at: https://www.neuroimaging.theclinics.com/
PET Clinics
Available at: https://www.pet.theclinics.com/

THE CLINICS ARE AVAILABLE ONLINE!
Access your subscription at:
www.theclinics.com

Contributors

CONSULTING EDITOR

SURESH K. MUKHERJI, MD, MBA, FACR
Professor, Department of Radiology, University of Louisville, Louisville, Kentucky, USA; Professor of Radiology, University of Illinois, Peoria, Illinois, USA; Professor, Department of Radiation Oncology, Robert Wood Johnson Medical School, Rutgers University, New Brunswick, New Jersey, USA; Faculty, Otolaryngology Head Neck Surgery, Michigan State University, Farmington Hills, Michigan, USA; National Director of Head and Neck Radiology, ProScan Imaging, Carmel, Indiana, USA

EDITORS

JOSEPH J. GEMMETE, MD, FACR, FSIR, FCIRSE, FAHA
Professor, Departments of Radiology, Neurosurgery, and Otolaryngology, Director, Neurointerventional Radiology Fellowship Program, Divisions of Neuroradiology, and Vascular and Interventional Radiology, Vascular/Interventional Radiologist and Neurointerventional Radiologist, Michigan Medicine, University of Michigan Hospitals, University of Michigan, Ann Arbor, Michigan, USA

ZACHARY M. WILSECK, MD
Clinical Assistant Professor, Division of Neuroradiology, Department of Radiology, Associate Program Director, Neurointerventional Radiology Fellowship, Medical Student and Resident Liaison, Neurointerventional Radiology, Neurointerventional Radiologist, Michigan Medicine, University of Michigan, Ann Arbor, Michigan, USA

AUTHORS

RAMEZ N. ABDALLA, MD, PhD
Assistant Professor, Department of Radiology, Northwestern University, Feinberg School of Medicine, Department of Radiology, Lurie Children's Hospital, Chicago, Illinois, USA; Department of Radiology, Ain Shams University, Faculty of Medicine, Egypt

MOHAMAD M. ALZEIN, BS
Department of Radiology, Northwestern University, Feinberg School of Medicine, Chicago, Illinois, USA

SAMEER A. ANSARI, MD, PhD
Professor, Department of Radiology, Northwestern University, Feinberg School of Medicine, Department of Radiology, Lurie Children's Hospital, Departments of Neurological Surgery and Neurology, Northwestern University, Feinberg School of Medicine, Chicago, Illinois, USA

MOMODOU Q. DAH, MPH
Michigan State University College of Human Medicine, Lansing, Michigan, USA

DONALD R. CANTRELL, MD, PhD
Assistant Professor, Department of Radiology, Northwestern University, Feinberg School of Medicine, Department of Radiology, Lurie Children's Hospital, Chicago, Illinois, USA

NEERAJ CHAUDHARY, MD
Clinical Professor, Departments of Neurosurgery, and Radiology, and Otorhinolaryngology, University of Michigan, Ann Arbor, Michigan, USA

HUANWEN CHEN, MD
Division of Interventional Neuroradiology,
Department of Diagnostic Radiology,
University of Maryland School of Medicine,
National Institute for Neurological Disorders
and Stroke, National Institutes of Health,
Bethesda, Maryland, USA; Department
of Neurology, MedStar Georgetown
University Hospital, Washington, DC,
USA

THOMAS L. CHENEVERT, PhD
Professor, Basic Radiological Sciences,
Department of Radiology, University of
Michigan, Ann Arbor, Michigan, USA

EPHRAIM CHURCH, MD, FAANS, FACS
Assistant Professor, Department of
Neurosurgery, Department of Neurosurgery,
and Department of Radiology, Penn State
Milton S. Hershey Medical Center, Hershey,
Pennsylvania, USA

MARCO COLASURDO, MD
Assistant Professor, Division of Interventional
Neuroradiology, Department of Diagnostic
Radiology, University of Maryland School of
Medicine, Baltimore, Maryland, USA;
Department of Interventional Radiology,
Oregon Health and Science University,
Portland, Oregon, USA

EHSAN DOLWATI, MD
Clinical Instructor, Department of
Neurosurgery, University of Michigan, Ann
Arbor, Michigan, USA

MAX FLEIGNER, BS
Oakland University, William Beaumont School
of Medicine, Detroit, Michigan, USA

CHANJU FRITCH, MD
Department of Neurosurgery, Penn State
Milton S. Hershey Medical Center, Hershey,
Pennsylvania, USA

DHEERAJ GANDHI, MBBS
Director, Division of Interventional
Neuroradiology, Professor of Department of
Diagnostic Radiology, University of Maryland
School of Medicine, Departments of Neurology
and Neurosurgery, University of Maryland
School of Medicine, Baltimore, Maryland,
USA

**JOSEPH J. GEMMETE, MD, FACR, FSIR,
FCIRSE, FAHA**
Professor, Departments of Radiology,
Neurosurgery, and Otolaryngology, Director,
Neurointerventional Radiology Fellowship
Program, Divisions of Neuroradiology, and
Vascular and Interventional Radiology,
Vascular/Interventional Radiologist and
Neurointerventional Radiologist, Michigan
Medicine, University of Michigan Hospitals,
University of Michigan, Ann Arbor, Michigan,
USA

ANDRES GUDINO-VEGA, MD
Department of Neurology, University of Iowa,
Iowa City, Iowa, USA

KATHERINE GUIJARRO-FALCON, MD
Department of Neurology, University of Iowa,
Iowa City, Iowa, USA

RICHARD KEEP, PhD
Professor, Department of Neurosurgery,
University of Michigan, Ann Arbor, Michigan,
USA

SRAVANTHI KODURI, MD
Chief Resident, Department of Neurosurgery,
University of Michigan, Ann Arbor, Michigan,
USA

LEANNE Y. LIN, MD, MPHS
Adjunct Clinical Instructor, Department of
Radiology, University of Michigan, Ann Arbor,
Michigan, USA

JACOB M. MILLER, BSE
Department of Neurology, University of Iowa,
Iowa City, Iowa, USA

LUIS E. NOBOA, BA
Universidad San Francisco de Quito, Quito,
Ecuador

ADITYA PANDEY, MD
Professor, Departments of Neurosurgery and
Radiology, University of Michigan, Ann Arbor,
Michigan, USA

SREEHARI PANICKER, MS
University of Michigan Medical School, Ann
Arbor, Michigan, USA

ABHINAV PATEL, MD
Department of Radiology, Northwestern
University, Feinberg School of Medicine,
Chicago, Illinois, USA

VENKATAKRISHNA RAJAJEE, MBBS
Clinical Professor, Departments of
Neurosurgery and Neurology, University of
Michigan, Ann Arbor, Michigan, USA

SAURABH ROHATGI, MD
Division of Neuroradiology, Department of
Radiology, Massachusetts General Hospital,
Harvard Medical School, Boston,
Massachusetts, USA

EDGAR A. SAMANIEGO, MD, MS
Clinical Associate Professor, Departments of
Neurology, Neurosurgery, and Radiology,
University of Iowa, Iowa City, Iowa, USA

SEBASTIAN SANCHEZ, MD
Department of Neurology, Yale University, New
Haven, Connecticut, USA

PAMELA W. SCHAEFER, MD
Diagnostic Radiologist, Division of
Neuroradiology, Professor, Department of
Radiology, Massachusetts General Hospital,
Harvard Medical School, Boston,
Massachusetts, USA

ALI SHAIBANI, MD
Professor, Department of Radiology,
Northwestern University, Feinberg School of
Medicine, Department of Radiology, Lurie
Children's Hospital, Department of Neurological
Surgery, Northwestern University, Feinberg
School of Medicine, Chicago, Illinois, USA

JONATHAN TROOST, PhD
Michigan Institute for Clinical and Health
Research, University of Michigan, Ann Arbor,
Michigan, USA

ANIL VASIREDDI, MD
Division of Neuroradiology, Department of
Radiology, Massachusetts General Hospital,
Harvard Medical School, Boston,
Massachusetts, USA

**DAVID ANDREW WILKINSON, MD, MS,
FAANS**
Assistant Professor, Department of
Neurosurgery, Penn State Milton S. Hershey
Medical Center, Hershey, Pennsylvania,
USA

ZACHARY M. WILSECK, MD
Clinical Assistant Professor, Division of
Neuroradiology, Department of Radiology,
Associate Program Director,
Neurointerventional Radiology Fellowship,
Medical Student and Resident Liaison,
Neurointerventional Radiology,
Neurointerventional Radiologist, Michigan
Medicine, University of Michigan, Ann Arbor,
Michigan, USA

GUOHUA XI, MD
Professor, Department of Neurosurgery,
University of Michigan, Ann Arbor, Michigan,
USA

Contents

> Computed tomography (CT), CT angiography (CTA), and CT perfusion (CTP) play
> crucial roles in the comprehensive evaluation and management of acute ischemic
> stroke, aneurysmal subarachnoid hemorrhage (SAH), and vasospasm. CTP provides
> functional data about cerebral blood flow, allowing radiologists, neurointerventional-
> ists, and stroke neurologists to more accurately delineate the volume of core infarct
> and ischemic penumbra allowing for patient-specific treatment decisions to be
> made. CTA and CTP are used in tandem to evaluate for vasospasm associated
> with aneurysmal SAH and can help provide an insight into the physiologic impact
> of angiographic vasospasm, better triaging patients for medical and interventional
> treatment.

> Ultrasound evaluation of the brain is performed through acoustic windows. Trans-
> cranial Doppler has long been used to monitor patients with subarachnoid hemor-
> rhage for cerebral vasospasm. Transcranial color-coded sonography permits
> parenchymal B-mode imaging and duplex evaluation. Transcranial ultrasound may
> also be used to assess the risk of delayed cerebral ischemia, screen patients for
> the presence of elevated intracranial pressure, confirm the diagnosis of brain death,
> measure midline shift, and detect ventriculomegaly. Transcranial ultrasound should
> be integrated with other point-of-care ultrasound techniques as an essential skill for
> the neurointensivist.

> Acute ischemic stroke (AIS) is a leading cause of death and disability worldwide, and
> its prevalence is expected to increase with global population aging and the burgeon-
> ing obesity epidemic. Clinical care for AIS has evolved during the past 3 decades,
> and it comprises of 3 major tenants: (1) timely recanalization of occluded vessels
> with intravenous thrombolysis or endovascular thrombectomy, (2) prompt initiation
> of antithrombotic agents to prevent stroke recurrences, and (3) poststroke suppor-
> tive care and rehabilitation. In this article, we summarize commonly used MR se-
> quences for AIS and DCI and highlight their clinical applications.

Momodou G. Bah, Ehsan Dolwati, Max Fleigner, Sravanthi Koduri, Aditya Pandey,
Leanne Y. Lin, Thomas L. Chenevert, Jonathan Troost, Guohua Xi, Richard Keep,
and Neeraj Chaudhary

This review article discusses the role of MR imaging-based biomarkers in understanding and managing hemorrhagic strokes, focusing on intracerebral hemorrhage
(ICH) and aneurysmal subarachnoid hemorrhage. ICH is a severe type of stroke with
high mortality and morbidity rates, primarily caused by the rupture of small blood
vessels in the brain, resulting in hematoma formation. MR imaging-based biomarkers, including brain iron quantification, ultra-early erythrolysis detection, and
diffusion tensor imaging, offer valuable insights for hemorrhagic stroke management. These biomarkers could improve early diagnosis, risk stratification, treatment
monitoring, and patient outcomes in the future, revolutionizing our approach to hemorrhagic strokes.

Sebastian Sanchez, Andres Gudino-Vega, Katherine Guijarro-Falcon, Jacob M. Miller,
Luis E. Noboa, and Edgar A. Samaniego

The evaluation of unruptured intracranial aneurysms requires a comprehensive and
multifaceted approach. The comprehensive analysis of aneurysm wall enhancement
through high-resolution MRI, in tandem with advanced processing techniques like
finite element analysis, quantitative susceptibility mapping, and computational fluid
dynamics, has begun to unveil insights into the intricate biology of aneurysms. This
enhanced understanding of the etiology, progression, and eventual rupture of aneurysms holds the potential to be used as a tool to triage patients to intervention versus
observation. Emerging tools such as radiomics and machine learning are poised to
contribute significantly to this evolving landscape of diagnostic refinement.

Joseph J. Gemmete

Dual-energy computed tomography (DECT) has emerged as a valuable imaging modality in the diagnosis and management of various cerebrovascular pathologies, including subarachnoid hemorrhage, intracranial hemorrhage, and acute ischemic
stroke. This article reviews the principles of DECT and its applications in the evaluation and management of these conditions. The author discuss the advantages of
DECT over conventional computed tomography, as well as its limitations, and provide an overview of current research and future directions in the field.

Mohamad M. Alzein, Abhinav Patel, Ramez N. Abdalla, Donald R. Cantrell, Ali Shaibani,
and Sameer A. Ansari

Conventional imaging modalities are utilized in evaluating intraluminal or intravascular pathology of the intracranial vessels. Limitations of luminal imaging techniques
can lead to inaccurate diagnosis, evaluation, and risk stratification, as many cerebrovascular pathologies involve the extrinsic vessel wall component. We attempt
to discuss the benefits of MRI based high-resolution vessel wall imaging, specifically

in the setting of intracranial atherosclerosis and vasculitis. In the setting of atherosclerosis, MR vessel wall imaging provides valuable diagnostic information regarding plaque location and characterization to predict ischemic stroke risk. Furthermore, it can provide information regarding the extent, treatment response, and biopsy targets for vasculitis cases.

 Video content accompanies this article at http://www.neuroimaging.theclinics.com.

Cerebrovascular surgery has many intraoperative imaging modalities available. Modern technologies include intraoperative digital subtraction angiogram, indocyanine green (ICG) angiography, relative fluorescent measurement with ICG, and ultrasound. Each of these can be used effectively in the treatment of open aneurysm and arteriovenous malformation surgeries, in addition to arteriovenous fistula surgery, and cerebral bypass surgery.

Acute stroke imaging plays a vital and time-sensitive role in therapeutic decision-making. Current clinical workflows widely use computed tomography (CT) and magnetic resonance (MR) techniques including CT and MR perfusion to estimate the volume of ischemic penumbra at risk for infarction without acute intervention. The use of imaging techniques aimed toward evaluating the metabolic derangements underlying a developing infarct may provide additional information for differentiating the penumbra from benign oligemia and infarct core. The authors review several modalities of metabolic imaging including PET, hydrogen and oxygen spectroscopy, sodium MRI, and pH-weighted MRI.

MR imaging's exceptional capabilities in vascular imaging stem from its ability to visualize and quantify vessel wall features, such as plaque burden, composition, and biomechanical properties. The application of advanced MR imaging techniques, including two-dimensional and three-dimensional black-blood MR imaging, T1 and T2 relaxometry, diffusion-weighted imaging, and dynamic contrast-enhanced MR imaging, wall shear stress, and arterial stiffness, empowers clinicians and researchers to explore the intricacies of vascular diseases. This array of techniques provides comprehensive insights into the development and progression of vascular pathologies, facilitating earlier diagnosis, targeted treatment, and improved patient outcomes in the management of vascular health.

Foreword

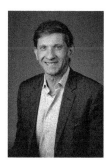

Suresh K. Mukherji, MD, MBA, FACR
Consulting Editor

Stroke continues to be a leading cause of morbidity and mortality. I am still amazed about the advancements made in stroke imaging over the past 30 years. I still remember as a resident looking at 10-mm slice thickness computed tomographic (CT) scans trying to determine if the small area of low attenuation in the basal ganglia was actually real or represented "quantum mottle." If we could convince ourselves (and others) it was "real," then we had to determine it was acute, subacute, or chronic.

My oh my…how things have changed since that time! The past three decades have seen incredible innovations in both invasive and noninvasive neuroimaging, which have improved early detection of stroke, successfully treated vessel occlusion, and improved outcomes. The pace of change continues to accelerate and makes it difficult to stay current with the latest advancements. It is with this in mind that we invited Drs Joseph Gemmete and Zachary Wilseck to Guest Edit this issue of *Neuroimaging Clinics* devoted to advanced imaging of hemorrhagic and ischemic stroke.

The issue begins with an overview of the pathophysiology of stroke and lays the foundation for more advanced topics. There are articles specifically devoted to transcranial ultrasound, numerous advanced CT (CT perfusion, dual-energy CT) and MR techniques (vessel wall imaging, MR biomarkers, quantitative MR images, spectroscopy). The articles are state-of-the-art and beautifully illustrated. The article authors are renowned experts in their fields, and I wish to personally thank each for their wonderful contributions.

Finally, I would like to thank Drs Gemmete and Wilseck for their efforts in creating such a wonderful issue of *Neuroimaging Clinics*. This contribution will certainly meet and exceed their goals of appealing to a wide multidisciplinary audience and improve patient care. On a personal note, I had the pleasure of working with Dr Gemmete when I was Neuroradiology Division Director at University Michigan. Joe was one of the most gifted interventionalists I have ever worked with, and I am so happy we are able to continue to collaborate.

DISCLOSURE

None.

Suresh K. Mukherji, MD, MBA, FACR
University of Louisville
Department of Radiology
530 S. Jackson Street, Suite C07
Louisville, KY, USA

E-mail address:
sureshmukherji@hotmail.com

Neuroimag Clin N Am 34 (2024) xv
https://doi.org/10.1016/j.nic.2024.02.004
1052-5149/24/© 2024 Published by Elsevier Inc.

neuroimaging.theclinics.com

Preface

Advanced Imaging of Hemorrhagic and Ischemic Stroke: The Future Holds Many Possibilities

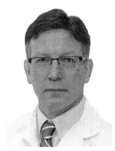
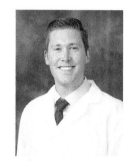

Joseph J. Gemmete, MD   Zachary M. Wilseck, MD
Editors

As we unveil this issue of *Neuroimaging Clinics*, dedicated to the nuanced realm of neurovascular imaging, our focus sharpens on the pivotal role it plays in diagnosing and managing hemorrhagic and ischemic strokes. This issue emerges at a time when the incidence of stroke continues to pose significant challenges to health care systems globally, underscoring the urgency for refined diagnostic capabilities and therapeutic strategies.

Stroke, a leading cause of mortality and enduring disability, presents a complex interplay of neurologic impairments that demand not only rapid and precise diagnostic approaches but also a deep understanding of the evolving landscape of neuroimaging techniques. The intent of this issue is to serve as a beacon, guiding clinicians and researchers through the intricacies of neurovascular imaging, with a keen emphasis on the latest innovations and their clinical implications in the context of hemorrhagic and ischemic stroke.

The journey of this issue begins with a foundational overview of the pathophysiology of stroke, setting the stage for a deeper exploration of the diverse imaging modalities at our disposal. From the established territories of computed tomography (CT) and MR imaging to the advancing frontiers of CT angiography, MR angiography, and perfusion imaging, each article is meticulously crafted to illuminate the strengths and limitations of these technologies in the acute and subacute phases of stroke management.

Our distinguished contributors, who are at the forefront of neuroimaging and cerebrovascular medicine, share their insights and experiences, weaving together a narrative that not only educates but also inspires. Their collective wisdom, distilled into this issue, aims to enhance the reader's proficiency in leveraging advanced imaging techniques to differentiate between hemorrhagic and ischemic strokes, thereby enabling more informed clinical decisions and tailored patient care.

Moreover, this issue acknowledges the dynamic nature of neurovascular disorders by including discussions on emerging therapeutic interventions and their imaging correlates. Understanding the interplay between novel treatments and neuroimaging findings is crucial for optimizing patient outcomes and advancing the field of stroke management.

The structure of the issue is intentionally designed to cater to a broad spectrum of readers, from seasoned experts in neuroimaging to clinicians and researchers endeavoring to deepen their understanding of neurovascular imaging. Through a blend of comprehensive reviews, cutting-edge research, and illustrative case studies, we aim to

Neuroimag Clin N Am 34 (2024) xvii–xviii
https://doi.org/10.1016/j.nic.2024.02.003
1052-5149/24/© 2024 Published by Elsevier Inc.

foster a holistic understanding of the current state and future directions of neurovascular imaging in the context of stroke.

In curating this issue, we have been privileged to collaborate with an array of esteemed authors, whose contributions reflect not only the depth of their expertise but also their commitment to improving patient care through innovation in neuroimaging. Their work, rigorous and enlightening, is a testament to the collaborative spirit that drives progress in medical science.

As you navigate through the articles of this issue, we hope you find both knowledge and inspiration. The field of neurovascular imaging is one of constant evolution, and it is through shared learning and collaboration that we can continue to improve the lives of those affected by stroke.

In closing, we extend our heartfelt gratitude to all contributors for their invaluable insights and to our readers, whose pursuit of excellence in clinical practice and research fuels the continuous advancement of neuroimaging. Together, we are not only witnesses to but also active participants in the unfolding narrative of neurovascular imaging and stroke medicine.

DISCLOSURES

The guest editors report no commercial or financial conflicts of interest or any funding sources.

Joseph J. Gemmete, MD
Michigan Medicine
University of Michigan Hospital
1500 East Medical Center Drive, UH B1D 330A
Ann Arbor, MI 48109-5030, USA

Zachary M. Wilseck, MD
Michigan Medicine
University of Michigan Hospital
1500 East Medical Center Drive, UHB1D530A
Ann Arbor, MI 48109-5030, USA

E-mail addresses:
gemmete@med.umich.edu (J.J. Gemmete)
zwilseck@med.umich.edu (Z.M. Wilseck)

CT Imaging Computed Tomography/Computed Tomography Angiography/Perfusion in Acute Ischemic Stroke and Vasospasm

Sreehari Panicker, MS[a,1], Zachary M. Wilseck, MD[b,*], Leanne Y. Lin, MD, MPHS[b,2], Joseph J. Gemmete, MD[b,c,d,3]

KEYWORDS

- CT angiography • CT perfusion • Acute ischemic stroke • Angiographic vasospasm
- Hemorrhagic stroke

KEY POINTS

- Computed tomography (CT), CT angiography (CTA), and CT perfusion (CTP) play crucial roles in the comprehensive evaluation and management of acute ischemic stroke (AIS), aneurysmal subarachnoid hemorrhage (SAH), and vasospasm.
- CTP provides functional data about cerebral blood flow, allowing radiologists, neurologists, and neurointerventionalists to more accurately delineate the volume of core infarct and ischemic penumbra allowing for patient-specific treatment decisions to be made.
- CTA and CTP are used in tandem to evaluate for vasospasm associated with aneurysmal SAH and can help provide an insight into the physiologic impact of angiographic vasospasm, better triaging patients for medical and interventional treatment.
- CT, CTA, and CTP provide a robust evaluation of AIS and hemorrhagic stroke, each contributing to a larger picture of the patient's cerebrovascular status, guiding immediate management and therapeutic strategies, and influencing prognosis.

INTRODUCTION

Neuroimaging plays a significant role in the assessment and diagnosis of patients in the setting of acute ischemic stroke (AIS) and hemorrhagic stroke. According to the World Health Organization,[1] stroke is the second most leading cause of death globally. Patients presenting with stroke-like symptoms often undergo imaging evaluation via noncontrast computed tomography (NCCT), computed tomography angiography (CTA), and/or computed tomography perfusion (CTP). While CT-based imaging remains the workhorse, other modalities including magnetic resonance imaging (MRI), magnetic resonance angiography (MRA), magnetic resonance perfusion (MRP), digital subtraction angiography (DSA), and transcranial Doppler may also have utility based on patient-specific pathology.

For patients presenting with AIS, CT imaging provides critical information used for guiding

[a] University of Michigan Medical School, Ann Arbor, MI, USA; [b] Department of Radiology, University of Michigan, Ann Arbor, MI 48109, USA; [c] Department of Neurosurgery, University of Michigan, Ann Arbor, MI 48109, USA; [d] Department of Otolaryngology, University of Michigan, Ann Arbor, MI 48109, USA
[1] Present address: 4038 Drexel Drive, Troy, MI 48098.
[2] Present address: 1020 North High Street, Unit 501, Columbus, OH 43201.
[3] Present address: 1500 East Medical Center Drive, B1D330A, Ann Arbor, MI 48109, USA
* Corresponding author. Department of Radiology, University of Michigan - Michigan Medicine, 1500 East Medical Center Drive, B1D530A, Ann Arbor, MI 48109.
E-mail address: zwilseck@med.umich.edu

Neuroimag Clin N Am 34 (2024) 175–189
https://doi.org/10.1016/j.nic.2024.01.004

treatment. For example, NCCT provides information regarding intracranial hemorrhage, which is a contraindication to thrombolysis. NCCT also allows for the evaluation of the degree of early ischemic changes, helping to guide possible reperfusion therapies. CTA allows for the identification of vessel occlusion and collateral status. CTP can provide information regarding infarct core size and surrounding hypoperfused, but at-risk brain tissue, termed ischemic penumbra.

In the setting of subarachnoid hemorrhage (SAH) and vasospasm, CTA and CTP play important roles in the identification of intracranial aneurysms, determining the severity of vasospasm, the vascular territories involved, and risk of ischemia. CTP can allow for the estimation of involved territories in the absence of reproducible clinical examination findings, evaluation of response to medical therapies, and help guide when intervention, including chemical or balloon angioplasty, may be indicated.

This article will outline these advanced imaging techniques, provide specific imaging protocols used in the setting of AIS and vasospasm related to hemorrhagic stroke, present case-based imaging examples, as well as pearls and pitfalls of CT, CTA, and CTP imaging.

COMPUTED TOMOGRAPHY
Background

CT is one of the initial imaging studies often used to evaluate patients who present with suspected stroke. The primary aim is to distinguish ischemic stroke from hemorrhagic stroke and other conditions that might present with similar symptoms, such as tumors or abscesses.

The key roles of CT in the evaluation of AIS are as follows:

Exclude hemorrhage
This is the most immediate purpose of a CT scan in a suspected stroke patient. A hemorrhagic stroke presents very differently on a CT scan compared with an ischemic stroke and has completely different management. It is crucial to rule this out before starting treatment, such as thrombolytic therapy, which can exacerbate bleeding.

Identify early signs of ischemia
In the acute phase (first few hours), an ischemic stroke may not be visible on a CT scan. However, with time, certain changes start to appear, such as loss of grey–white differentiation, hypoattenuation, or localized brain swelling. However, these signs often become apparent several hours after the onset of symptoms.

Detect large vessel occlusion
While CTA is used to visualize the blood vessels in the brain and neck, NCCT can identify a "hyperdense vessel sign," focal hyperdensity within a large vessel secondary to thromboembolic material within the lumen. This may be the earliest visible sign of ischemic stroke.

Evaluate for infarct size and location
A CT scan can help to identify the location and extent of an ischemic stroke, which can aid in prognostication and guide management decisions. The Alberta Stroke Program Early CT Score (ASPECTS) is a 10-point score allowing for quantitative evaluation of ischemic changes. This involves the evaluation of the bilateral caudate, putamen, internal capsule, and insular cortex along with 3 areas of the middle cerebral artery territory at both the ganglionic level and supraganglionic level (6 areas total). One point is deducted from 10 for every region involved. Initial data showed that patients with an ASPECTS of 7 or lesser had the worse functional outcomes at 3 months and an increased risk of hemorrhage.[2] Variations of the ASPECTS system have been created for the evaluation of posterior circulation infarcts, referred to as pc-ASPECTS.[3]

Detect contraindications to therapy
Some patients may have conditions that are contraindications to certain therapies. For example, evidence of a recent hemorrhage, large areas of established infarction, or certain types of tumors may be contraindications to thrombolytic therapy.

While a CT scan is a crucial diagnostic tool in the evaluation of AIS, it is important to note that it is just one part of the evaluation process. Clinical assessment, including a thorough history and neurologic examination, is also essential. Additionally, other diagnostic tools may also be used, such as MR imaging, which can be more sensitive than CT for detecting small or early infarcts, particularly in the posterior fossa.

COMPUTED TOMOGRAPHY ANGIOGRAPHY
Background

Computed tomography angiography (CTA) has become a critical component in the assessment of AIS. It offers a detailed and noninvasive view of the cerebral vasculature, allowing for the prompt identification of large vessel occlusions (LVOs), evaluation of collateral circulation, and the detection of potential sources of emboli. Moreover, CTA plays a pivotal role in detecting and monitoring cerebral aneurysms and vasospasm, critical components of stroke care related to SAH. Speed, availability, and accuracy have made CTA a cornerstone of stroke imaging, impacting therapeutic decisions and patient outcomes.

Protocol

CTA entails multiple key considerations including field of view, bolus tracking, timing, and other relevant parameters to maximize its diagnostic accuracy.

CTA is performed by injecting an iodine-based contrast material intravenously while imaging the head and/or cervical vasculature utilizing CT. Patients are typically scanned in the supine position, and the images are usually acquired in a caudal-cranial direction following the administration of the contrast (some older scanners can utilize a cranial-caudal direction to minimize venous contamination in the head portion of the scan). The scan is typically performed in a helical mode with thin slices (0.5–1.0 mm), which are subsequently reconstructed into thicker slabs for interpretation. Thin-slice acquisition is crucial for capturing small vascular details such as aneurysms, vasospasm, or arterial dissections.[4]

The dose of contrast and the rate of injection can vary per institutional protocol, but typically, a dose of 60 to 80 mL of contrast (around 300–370 mg of iodine/mL) at a rate of 3 to 5 mL/s is used to achieve appropriate opacification of vessels followed by saline flush. The timing of the scan relative to the contrast administration is a critical factor to consider. Techniques such as bolus tracking or test bolus may be used to optimize this timing. In bolus tracking, a region of interest (ROI) is placed in a vessel (often the proximal descending aorta), and imaging begins once the contrast enhancement in the ROI reaches a certain threshold (ex: 120 HU). The test bolus method involves injecting a small amount of contrast and performing a time–density curve to determine the optimal delay time for the main acquisition.[5]

Some protocols may incorporate multiphase CTA, which involves acquiring additional scans at later time points (eg, 30 seconds and 60 seconds after the initial scan). This technique can provide valuable information about the dynamics of blood flow, particularly useful in the setting of AIS, where it can highlight regions of delayed perfusion and can also offer additional opportunities to visualize vasospasm, aneurysms, and importantly collateral flow.[6]

Finally, the images obtained are often postprocessed using multiplanar reformatting (MPR) and 3-dimensional reconstructions, which can help visualize complex vascular structures and can improve the detection of aneurysms and vasospasm.[7]

Interpreting Computed Tomography Angiography Images

Images should be reviewed in a systematic fashion to minimize the likelihood of perceptual error, the most common cause of radiologic error in image interpretation. The radiologist is assessing the following:

Extracranial vessels
The extracranial vasculature must be thoroughly evaluated from the caudal-most included aspect to the skull base. It is important to evaluate the aortic configuration and origins of the cervical vasculature to identify anomalous courses, ostial stenosis, or occlusion. The cervical vasculature must also be evaluated for any significant stenosis, dissection, or occlusion, particularly in the carotid and vertebral arteries. The degree of vascular stenosis is typically classified based on the North American Symptomatic Carotid Endarterectomy Trial criteria.

Intracranial vessels
The circle of Willis and its branches must be meticulously evaluated. Each branch should be followed out as distally as possible. Multiplanar reconstruction (MPR) and maximum intensity projection (MIP) images should also be evaluated to increase the sensitivity of identifying both large and medium vessel occlusions (Fig. 1). Other vascular features including luminal narrowing and luminal irregularity should also be noted, as they could suggest vasculitis, dissection, or vasospasm in the proper clinical settings. Aneurysms classically present as focal outpouchings of the vessels, most commonly located at vessel bifurcation or branch points; however, fusiform or blister type aneurysms can sometimes be more difficult to identify and can occur anywhere along the vessel course.

Collateral flow
Note the presence and extent of collateral flow, as robust collaterals may help to maintain perfusion to the ischemic tissue and slow the rate of infarct progression.

Vascular anomalies
Arteriovenous malformations or other vascular anomalies including dural arteriovenous fistulae can result in seizures, headaches, focal neurologic deficits, or other stroke mimickers. Dependent on contrast bolus timing, there may be adequate opacification of the venous structures, which can allow for the evaluation of the dural venous sinuses and cortical veins for thrombosis.

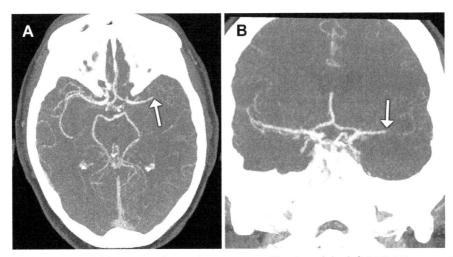

Fig. 1. Axial (*A*) and coronal (*B*) MIP CTA shows abrupt nonopacification of the left MCA M1 segment (*arrow*).

Soft tissues

The soft tissues of the head and neck must be thoroughly evaluated. Incidental head and neck masses, lymphadenopathy, thyroid lesions, or even lung cancers must be identified as this data can inform clinicians about potential etiologies of AIS.

Pitfalls

There are several potential pitfalls when interpreting CTA in acute stroke.

Beam hardening artifacts

Dense structures, such as bone or calcified plaques, can create artifacts that might mimic or obscure a vessel occlusion.

Timing of contrast

If the scan is performed too early or too late relative to the contrast administration, it can result in suboptimal opacification of the vessels and hinder accurate interpretation.

Vessel mimics

Nonvascular structures can sometimes mimic vascular pathology. For example, hypodense structures such as the subarachnoid spaces can mimic vessel occlusion (the "pseudo-occlusion" phenomenon).

Underestimation of the infarct core

CTA provides information about the vascular anatomy but does not directly image the brain tissue. Consequently, it might underestimate the extent of infarction, especially in the early stages. For a more accurate estimation, CTP or diffusion-weighted MR imaging should be considered.

Underestimation of aneurysms and vasospasm

Small aneurysms or mild vasospasm may not be adequately visualized on CTA, particularly when limited by beam hardening artifact related to nearby bone and metal (coils, stents, and clips). In certain instances, CTA may fail to depict the true neck/dome/adjacent small vessel anatomy. Further diagnostic evaluation may be necessary if clinical suspicion remains high.[8]

Overall, CTA is an essential part of modern acute stroke care. It provides key information that can guide therapy and predict outcomes. Nonetheless, like any imaging modality, it must be interpreted in the context of the overall clinical picture.

COMPUTED TOMOGRAPHY PERFUSION
Background

CT perfusion has revolutionized the field of medical imaging, notably within the realm of AIS management. This noninvasive imaging modality has transitioned from a research tool to a crucial clinical instrument for diagnosing and managing ischemic stroke, while changing how health care professionals assess cerebrovascular pathology and treatment options.

CTP allows clinicians to visualize cerebral hemodynamics, providing quantifiable measures of cerebral perfusion. Cerebral blood flow (CBF) is the volume of blood (mL) per 100 g of brain tissue per minute, cerebral blood volume (CBV) is the volume of blood (mL) per 100 g of brain tissue, mean transit time (MTT) is the average time it takes blood to pass through a given region, time-to-peak (TTP) perfusion is the time for blood to reach peak perfusion. By mapping these parameters, physicians gain insights into the location and extent of ischemic brain tissue, thus enabling personalized treatment strategies and potentially improving patient outcomes.

Before the advent of CTP, the management of AIS was largely guided by the time since symptom onset, a strategy that often fell short of capturing the heterogeneity of patient conditions. CTP allows for the physiologic evaluation of cerebral tissue to estimate areas of infarction and areas with hypoperfusion that are at risk for infarction (penumbra). CTP has also been proven critical in the detection of delayed cerebral ischemia (DCI) following aneurysmal SAH and vasospasm. By identifying areas of reduced cerebral flow and increased MTT, CTP can aid in the early detection of vasospasm even before clinical symptoms manifest.[9]

With the introduction of CTP, stroke treatment moved from a time-based paradigm to a tissue-based paradigm.

Protocol

The acquisition of CTP images is a process that incorporates patient preparation, a properly designed scanning protocol, and the administration of an iodinated contrast agent. Each step of this process needs to be carefully calibrated to yield accurate and clinically useful results. The objective of CTP imaging is to generate a time–density curve reflecting the passage of contrast through the cerebral vasculature and from this data derive vital parameters such as CBF, CBV, and MTT.

To begin, the patient is positioned within the CT scanner gantry, often in the supine position with the head secured to minimize movement. The area of the brain to be imaged—typically a 4 to 16-cm segment at the level of the basal ganglia—is then selected. The coverage may vary depending on the scanner's capabilities and the clinical context; newer multidetector CT scanners can allow for coverage of the entire brain.

Next, a bolus of iodinated contrast agent is administered intravenously, usually in the antecubital vein. The contrast dosage and injection rate are determined based on the patient's body weight and kidney function to ensure optimal enhancement while minimizing risks. Typical protocols recommend a contrast volume of 40 to 50 mL at an injection rate of 4 to 5 mL/s, followed by a saline flush to clear the contrast from the veins and reduce streak artifacts.[10]

Once the contrast injection is initiated, a rapid series of low-dose CT scans is performed, typically beginning a few seconds after the start of the contrast injection to allow time for the contrast to reach the cerebral circulation. This sequence continues for 45 to 60 seconds to capture the peak enhancement of the brain parenchyma and the clearance of the contrast. The precise timing can vary based on factors such as the patient's cardiac output and the scanner's capabilities.

The scanning protocol, including the slice thickness, rotation time, tube current, and tube voltage, is optimized to balance image quality with radiation dose. The protocol may also be adjusted for specific clinical scenarios; for example, in a patient with a suspected high-grade stenosis or occlusion, a delay in image acquisition may be necessary to account for the slower passage of contrast.

The acquisition of CTP images is a dynamic process requiring rapid data acquisition, precise timing, and meticulous patient care. While it provides invaluable information about cerebral perfusion, it is not without its challenges. As noted by Sanelli and colleagues,[11] differences in acquisition protocols and contrast administration can introduce variability in perfusion measurements. There is also an inherent risk of patient movement during the scan, which can lead to motion artifacts.

Postprocessing of Computed Tomography Perfusion

Postprocessing of CTP images is a vital step to extract cerebral hemodynamic parameters. This process transforms the raw CTP data, a series of images showing the distribution of contrast over time, into color-coded maps that can be visually and quantitatively interpreted.

Once the CTP data is acquired, it undergoes several stages of postprocessing, including motion correction, noise reduction, arterial input function (AIF), and venous output function selection. Following these initial steps, the key aspect of postprocessing is the application of a mathematical model to generate the perfusion maps. The 2 most used models are the deconvolution-based and the maximum slope models.[12]

The deconvolution-based model applies a mathematical process called deconvolution to the time–density curves obtained from the CTP data, creating maps of CBF, CBV, and MTT. This model is robust and generally considered more accurate for determining MTT, but it is computationally intensive and may be sensitive to noise.

In contrast, the maximum slope model calculates perfusion parameters based on the maximum slope of the time–density curve, which represents the fastest rate of contrast arrival and clearance. While this model is simpler and faster, it may be less accurate, particularly in conditions with altered hemodynamics, such as high-grade stenosis or collateral circulation.[12]

The created perfusion maps undergo color-coding to visually depict the perfusion status of the brain tissue. Typically, areas of reduced CBF and increased MTT with preservation or increased CBV suggest penumbra, while areas with prolongation of MTT and TTP and decreased CBV and CBF indicate infarct core. Areas of decreased CBV roughly correspond to core infarct volume. Still, interpretation can be complex, as these parameters can be influenced by numerous factors, including the choice of postprocessing software and the selected AIF.[13]

Postprocessing of CTP images also includes the generation of maps showing the ischemic penumbra and infarct core. Differences or "mismatch" between the volume of penumbra and infarct core can be crucial for treatment decision-making in AIS[14] (Figs. 2 and 3).

While the postprocessing of CTP data provides invaluable insights into cerebral perfusion, challenges exist. Different software packages use different mathematical models and algorithms, leading to potential variability in the derived perfusion parameters. This variability can make it difficult to establish universal thresholds for the ischemic core and penumbra.[13]

Moreover, postprocessing can be time-consuming, which can be a significant constraint in the acute stroke setting. Advances in automated and artificial intelligence (AI)-based postprocessing techniques are promising solutions to this challenge and the subject of ongoing research.[15]

Software Packages

Postprocessing of CTP images is essential for translating the raw data into quantifiable and visually interpretable maps of cerebral perfusion. Various software packages are available for this purpose, each with its unique algorithms, features, and potential benefits. The choice of software can influence the derived perfusion parameters and, therefore, clinical decision-making. Some of the most used CTP postprocessing software packages include the following:

1. Philips IntelliSpace Portal: This comprehensive software package from Philips Healthcare (Cambridge, MA) includes a suite of advanced visualization and analysis tools, including CTP postprocessing. The software provides maps of CBF, CBV, and MTT, as well as TTP and delay maps.
2. RAPID.AI: Developed by iSchemaView (Golden, CO), RAPID.AI is a fully automated postprocessing software for CTP, as well as MRP and diffusion. It provides color-coded maps of CBF, CBV, MTT, and the ischemic core and penumbra. RAPID.AI is recognized for its role in several landmark clinical trials, including DEFUSE 3 and DAWN.
3. Olea Sphere: Provided by Olea Medical (La Ciotat, France), Olea Sphere offers a range of advanced imaging postprocessing tools, including CTP analysis. The software provides standard CTP maps (CBF, CBV, and MTT) and includes features such as automated arterial and venous input function selection and motion correction.
4. Siemens syngo.via: Siemens' syngo.via (Malvern, PA) platform includes a comprehensive CTP analysis module that provides the standard perfusion maps and allows for customizable thresholds and ROI selection. It also includes features for automatic skull stripping and motion correction.
5. GE AW Server: GE's (Chicago, IL) Advanced Workstation Server includes a suite of postprocessing applications, including CTP analysis. The software provides color-coded perfusion maps and includes features such as automatic vessel detection and ROI analysis.
6. Viz.ai: Viz.ai (San Francisco, CA) is a fully automated postprocessing software for CTP, as well as MRP and diffusion. It provides color-

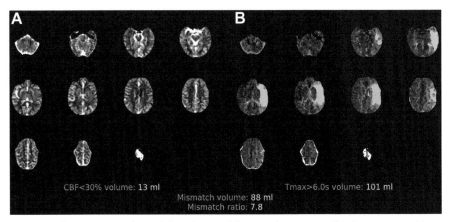

CBF<30% volume: 13 ml   Tmax>6.0s volume: 101 ml
Mismatch volume: 88 ml
Mismatch ratio: 7.8

Fig. 2. CTP automated postprocessed CBF (A) and Tmax (B) maps shows a small infarct core and large region of ischemic penumbra.

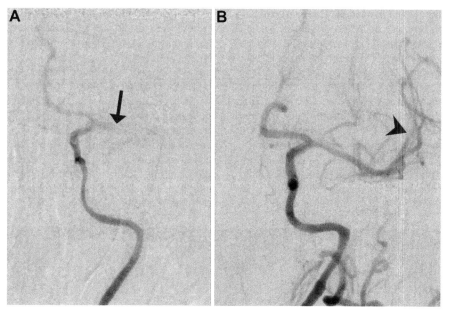

Fig. 3. Prethrombectomy AP projection angiography (*A*) confirmed the occlusion (*arrow*), which was treated with thrombectomy. Postthrombectomy angiography (*B*) shows successful recanalization of the vessel with visualization of distal branches (*arrowhead*).

coded maps of CBF, CBV, MTT, and the ischemic core and penumbra.

Each of these software packages has its strengths and potential limitations, and the choice of software may depend on a variety of factors, including the specific clinical scenario, the CT scanner used, the institution's protocols, and the physician's preference and familiarity with the software.

It is worth noting that ongoing advances in AI and machine learning are leading to the development of new software tools for CTP postprocessing. These tools aim to automate and streamline the postprocessing workflow, improve the accuracy and consistency of perfusion parameter estimation, and potentially provide new insights into cerebral perfusion and the ischemic process.

Interpreting Computed Tomography Perfusion Images

Interpreting CTP images is a critical task that provides essential information about the CBF, CBV, and MTT, helping guide the management of patients with AIS. However, this task requires careful attention to both the qualitative and quantitative aspects of the perfusion maps, as well as an understanding of the potential limitations and pitfalls.

CTP generates several color-coded maps, including CBF, CBV, and MTT maps, which provide information about different aspects of cerebral perfusion.

- CBF: This map represents the volume of blood flowing through a given amount of brain tissue per unit time. Areas of significantly reduced CBF may represent ischemic or infarcted tissue. In the context of an AIS, a region with a markedly reduced CBF compared with the surrounding tissue is typically indicative of the ischemic core, which represents tissue that has already suffered irreversible damage.
- CBV: This map reflects the total volume of blood in a given amount of brain tissue. In AIS, a region with significantly decreased CBV is also indicative of the ischemic core, the irreversibly damaged tissue. It is noteworthy that the CBV map is particularly helpful to distinguish the infarct core from the penumbra (ischemic but potentially salvageable tissue).
- MTT: This map shows the average time it takes for blood to pass through a given amount of brain tissue. Areas with significantly prolonged MTT may indicate impaired perfusion due to a reduced blood supply, such as in the setting of a stroke. Regions of prolonged MTT but preserved CBF and CBV suggest the ischemic penumbra, the area of brain tissue that is at risk of infarction but potentially salvageable with prompt reperfusion therapy.

In addition to these maps, some software packages generate a TTP map, showing the time it takes for the contrast to reach its peak concentration within the tissue. This map can also help identify areas of delayed perfusion.

The concept of the ischemic penumbra is fundamental to interpreting CTP images in AIS and cerebral vasospasm. The ischemic penumbra is the region of brain tissue that is at risk of infarction but potentially salvageable. On CTP, this region is typically represented by an area of reduced CBF and prolonged MTT but preserved CBV. In contrast, the ischemic core shows reductions in all 3 parameters. Identifying the penumbra is critical for treatment decisions, as patients with a significant penumbra may benefit from reperfusion therapies (Figs. 4–6).

The early detection and management of DCI is central to determining functional outcomes among patients with SAH.[16] There is a notable discrepancy where vessel narrowing seen on conventional imaging (CTA) is not always correlated with the development of neurologic deficits from DCI.[17] The CBF maps generated by CTP can show microcirculatory dysfunction not seen on CT, CTA, or DSA, further revealing ischemic tissue downstream of a large vessel with vasospasm. This can be particularly useful when evaluating for DCI amid the multiple confounding factors (fever, metabolic alterations, infection, and rebleeding) contributing to clinical deterioration after SAH[18] (Fig. 7).

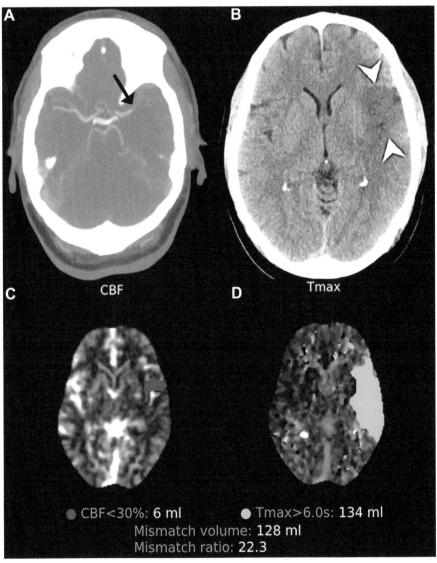

Fig. 4. Outside institution, axial MIP CTA (*A*) reveals an abrupt occlusion of the left M1 segment and axial non-contrast CT (*B*) shows loss of the gray–white differentiation in the left insula and opercula (*arrowheads*). The CTP reveals an estimated core infarct of 6 mL (*C*) and ischemic penumbra mismatch volume of 128 mL (*D*). *Black arrow* is at the point of abrupt occlusion of the left M1 segment.

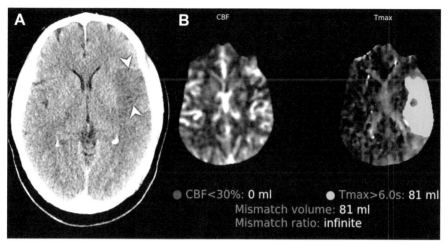

A

B CBF   Tmax

● CBF<30%: **0 ml**   ● Tmax>6.0s: **81 ml**
Mismatch volume: **81 ml**
Mismatch ratio: **infinite**

Fig. 5. Upon transfer to our hospital, noncontrast CT (*A*) appears unchanged with a similar loss of the gray–white matter differentiation in the left insula and opercula (*arrowheads*); however, CTP (*B*) reveals the estimated core and ischemic penumbra volumes have decreased to 0 mL and 81 mL respectively, suspected to represent pseudonormalization.

However, the interpretation of CTP images is not without its challenges. The perfusion parameters can be influenced by numerous factors, including patient-specific factors (eg, cardiac output, blood pressure), technical factors (eg, contrast timing, injection rate), and postprocessing factors (eg, selection of the AIF, deconvolution algorithm). Understanding these factors and how they can impact the perfusion maps is crucial for accurate interpretation.

Moreover, while there are general thresholds for the perfusion parameters that indicate the ischemic core and penumbra, these can vary based on the specific clinical and imaging context. Therefore, CTP interpretation should always be performed in conjunction with other clinical and imaging information.

Caveats and Pitfalls

While CTP imaging has revolutionized the diagnosis and management of AIS and helped guide the medical and endovascular treatment of cerebral vasospasm and DCI, several caveats and pitfalls must be considered during image acquisition, postprocessing, and interpretation to ensure accurate results. These limitations encompass technical aspects, patient factors, and interpretative challenges, all of which can significantly impact clinical decision-making.

1. Technical considerations: The quality of CTP data is highly dependent on technical aspects of the scan, including contrast bolus timing, injection rate, and scan duration. Incorrect timing of the contrast bolus can lead to underestimation

or overestimation of perfusion parameters, leading to potential misinterpretation.[19] Additionally, if the scan duration is too short, it may not adequately capture the passage of contrast, leading to inaccuracies in the perfusion maps.[20]

2. Patient factors: Perfusion parameters can be influenced by patient-specific factors, such as cardiac output and blood pressure, potentially leading to inaccurate estimation of the ischemic core and penumbra. Moreover, patients with poor renal function or acute kidney injury may be at risk for contrast-induced nephropathy, limiting the use of CTP in this population.[21]

3. Postprocessing challenges: The postprocessing of CTP data, including the selection of the AIF and the application of the deconvolution algorithm, can significantly impact the derived perfusion parameters. Different software packages use different algorithms and have varying degrees of user-defined inputs, leading to potential variability in the perfusion maps.[13]

4. Interpretative challenges: The interpretation of CTP images requires a careful understanding of cerebral hemodynamics and the technical aspects of CTP. Thresholds for the ischemic core and penumbra can vary, and these areas can evolve over time, complicating the interpretation.[20] Furthermore, areas of "matched" low CBF and CBV can reflect either the ischemic core or benign oligemia, leading to potential overestimation of the infarct core.[19]

5. Radiation dose: While newer techniques and protocols have significantly reduced radiation

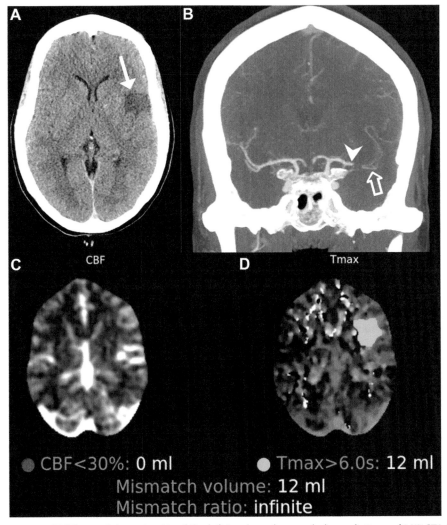

Fig. 6. Noncontrast CT (*A*) reveals hypodensity of the left insula and opercula (*arrow*). Coronal MIP CTA (*B*) reveals occlusion of the mid to distal left M1 segment (*arrowhead*) with distal reconstitution (*open arrow*). CTP reveals a small estimated ischemic penumbra (*D*), however no core infarct (*C*), even though there was a clear region of hypodensity on noncontrast CT, suspected to represent pseudonormalization.

exposure, CTP imaging still involves ionizing radiation, which can be a concern, particularly in young patients and those who require repeated scans.[22]

Despite these challenges, CTP remains a critical tool for the management of AIS and vasospasm evaluation. Ongoing advances in CTP techniques, postprocessing algorithms, and interpretation strategies continue to improve the accuracy and utility of this imaging modality.

When applied for the evaluation of cerebral vasospasm, CTP bears an additional caveat: Statistical variance. When evaluating the severity of vasospasm, different perfusion maps have demonstrated various levels of diagnostic accuracy in detecting vasospasm. Temporal perfusion

(MTT and time to drain [TTD]) maps yield higher levels of accuracy with TTD yielding the highest sensitivity in correlating to angiography of discovering existing vasospasm.[23]

Limitations in Differentiating Normal from Pathologic Tissue

The differentiation of normal from pathologic tissue is an essential component of CTP imaging, particularly in the context of AIS and vasospasm. However, there are several limitations in this differentiation process.

1. Benign oligemia: This is a condition where there is decreased CBF, but not to the extent that it causes tissue damage. It can be challenging

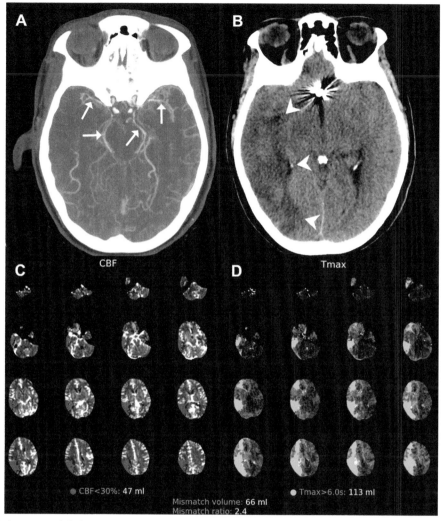

Fig. 7. Axial CTA MIP (A) shows a beaded appearance of the bilateral MCAs and PCAs, worse on the right (*arrows*). This correlates with the noncontrast CT (B) showing hypodensity and loss of grey–white differentiation in the right cerebral hemisphere (*arrowheads*). CTP (C) shows a large region of slow perfusion and small estimated core infarct (D).

to differentiate benign oligemia from true ischemic penumbra, as both can show reduced CBF on CTP. However, benign oligemia is not at immediate risk of infarction and does not benefit from reperfusion therapies. Misinterpretation can lead to overestimation of the penumbra and unnecessary interventions.[19]

2. Ischemic core estimation: The accurate delineation of the ischemic core, the irreversibly damaged tissue, is essential for therapeutic decisions. However, there is significant variability in the thresholds used to define the core on CTP, leading to potential inaccuracies in core estimation.[20]

3. Microvascular obstruction: In some cases, microvascular obstruction can cause regions

of reduced CBF and CBV that mimic the ischemic core on CTP. However, these regions can potentially be reperfused and do not represent true irreversible infarction.[24]

4. Collateral flow: Good collateral flow can maintain CBF and CBV in the ischemic territory, leading to underestimation of the penumbra on CTP. The absence of collateral flow can also overestimate the ischemic core, as it may reduce perfusion in areas not directly supplied by the occluded vessel.[14]

5. Effect of patient factors: Individual patient factors such as cardiac output, blood pressure, and hematocrit levels can impact perfusion parameters and influence the differentiation of normal from pathologic tissue.[25]

6. Postprocessing and interpretative variability: Differences in postprocessing algorithms, the selection of AIF, and interpretative variability can lead to discrepancies in the delineation of normal and pathologic tissue.[13]

Thus, while CTP imaging provides invaluable insights into cerebral perfusion, careful consideration of these limitations is essential for accurate differentiation of normal from pathologic tissue and appropriate clinical decision-making.

Clinical Use–Mismatch Concept

The clinical use of CTP imaging in AIS has been greatly enhanced by the development of the "mismatch concept." This concept involves comparing areas of the brain with compromised blood flow (hypoperfusion, representing the ischemic penumbra or "tissue at risk") to areas of irreversibly damaged tissue (ischemic core), to identify patients who may benefit from reperfusion therapies.[26]

1. Ischemic core: This is the region of brain tissue where the blood flow has been sufficiently reduced to cause irreversible damage. On CTP, the ischemic core is typically identified by significantly reduced CBF and CBV.[20]
2. Penumbra (tissue at risk): The penumbra is the region surrounding the ischemic core where the blood flow is reduced but not to the extent that it causes immediate cell death. It is considered "tissue at risk" as it can potentially progress to infarction if not promptly reperfused. On CTP, the penumbra is usually identified by reduced CBF but normal or increased CBV.[20]
3. Mismatch concept: The mismatch concept postulates that patients with a large "mismatch"—a large area of penumbra (or tissue at risk) compared to a small core—are most likely to benefit from reperfusion therapies, as they have a substantial amount of salvageable brain tissue. Conversely, patients with a "matched" defect (ie, the core and penumbra are approximately the same size) are less likely to benefit from reperfusion therapies, as most of the affected tissue is already irreversibly damaged.[26]

The mismatch concept forms the basis for patient selection in several recent clinical trials of endovascular therapy for AIS, such as the DEFUSE 3 and DAWN trials. These trials demonstrated improved outcomes in patients with a favorable mismatch profile who were treated up to 24 hours from symptom onset, thus expanding the therapeutic window for AIS.[27,28]

However, the application of the mismatch concept in clinical practice requires careful interpretation, considering the limitations and potential pitfalls of CTP imaging, including variability in threshold values for the ischemic core and penumbra, the differentiation of benign oligemia from true penumbra, and the influence of collateral flow on perfusion parameters.[14,19]

Predicting Response to Reperfusion

CTP imaging plays a critical role in predicting the response to treatment in patients with AIS. By providing real-time information about cerebral perfusion and the extent of ischemic injury, CTP can help identify patients who may benefit from reperfusion therapies and those who may be at risk of harmful effects such as hemorrhagic transformation. The following are some key points to consider:

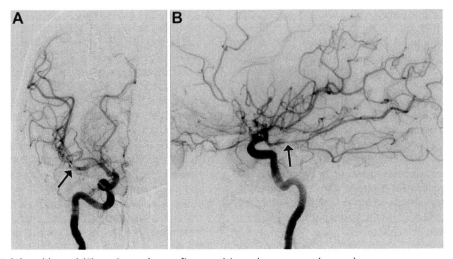

Fig. 8. AP (A) and lateral (B) angiography confirms multivessel vasospasm (arrows).

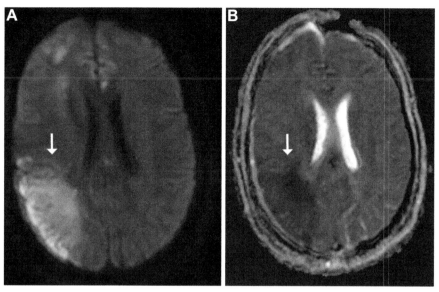

Fig. 9. Diffusion-weighted images (*A*) and apparent diffusion map (*B*) on MR imaging confirms regions of infarct (*arrows*).

1. Perfusion-diffusion mismatch: CTP can help to predict the response to treatment by identifying a "mismatch" between the volume of tissue with compromised blood flow and the core of infarcted tissue (Figs. 4–7). Patients with a significant mismatch, indicating a large volume of salvageable tissue, are considered good candidates for reperfusion therapies such as thrombolysis or thrombectomy. The DEFUSE 3 and DAWN trials demonstrated improved outcomes in these patients, even when treated up to 24 hours from symptom onset.[27,28]

2. Collateral circulation: The presence and quality of collateral circulation, which can be evaluated on CTP, have been shown to influence the response to treatment. Patients with good collateral circulation are more likely to have smaller infarct cores, larger volumes of salvageable tissue, and better clinical outcomes after reperfusion therapies.[14]

3. TTP maps: The extent of delay on TTP maps has been found to correlate with the clinical outcome in patients undergoing reperfusion therapies. A large delay (>6 seconds) on TTP maps may predict a poor response to therapy and an increased risk of hemorrhagic transformation.[29]

However, the prediction of treatment response based on CTP must consider the limitations and potential pitfalls of this imaging modality, including variability in threshold values for the ischemic core and penumbra, and the influence of patient and technical factors on perfusion parameters.[20]

CTP has reshaped the landscape of acute stroke management. Despite its inherent limitations, its pivotal role in delineating the ischemic core and penumbra, and thereby guiding treatment strategies, cements its position in the clinical toolbox.

SUMMARY

In conclusion, CT, CTA, and CTP play crucial roles in the comprehensive evaluation and management of AIS, aneurysmal SAH, and vasospasm. Each modality provides unique and complementary information that assists clinicians in making critical treatment decisions.

NCCT scans are often the first step in neurologic imaging, being readily available, fast, and effective in distinguishing ischemic stroke from hemorrhagic stroke. It can show early signs of ischemia such as loss of grey–white differentiation and localized parenchymal edema as well as identify the distribution and degree of SAH and its possible sequela including hydrocephalus. NCCT can guide clinicians in identifying indications or contraindications for certain therapies.

CTA expands on this by offering a detailed view of the cerebral vasculature. In ischemic stroke, this allows for the identification of LVOs, evaluation of collateral circulation, and detection of potential sources of emboli. In the setting of aneurysmal SAH, CTA allows for the identification of intracranial aneurysms and the detection of vasospasm. This information is crucial as it can directly impact therapeutic decisions, such as the consideration of endovascular treatment.

CTP further enhances the evaluation by providing functional data about CBF. This can help delineate the extent of the core infarct from the penumbra (the area of brain tissue that is at risk but not yet infarcted), assisting in the selection of patients who may benefit from acute interventions even beyond the conventional time windows (Figs. 8 and 9).

In concert, these imaging modalities provide a robust evaluation of AIS and hemorrhagic stroke, each contributing to a larger picture of the patient's cerebrovascular status, guiding immediate management and therapeutic strategies, and influencing prognosis. It is important, however, to interpret their findings in the context of the overall clinical scenario, considering the patient's symptoms, medical history, and physical examination. A comprehensive, multidimensional approach is crucial in the management of acute ischemic and hemorrhagic stroke to ensure the best possible patient outcomes.

CLINICS CARE POINTS

- CT, CTA, and CTP play crucial roles in the comprehensive evaluation and management of AIS, aneurysmal SAH, and vasospasm.
- NCCT is the first step in stroke imaging as it is readily available, fast, and effective and distinguishing ischemic stroke from hemorrhagic stroke.
- CTA offers a detailed evaluation of the cerebral vasculature allowing for the detection of large vessel occlusion, intracranial aneurysms, vasospasm, and vascular malformations.
- CTP provides functional data regarding cerebral blood flow, further assisting in the selection of patients who may benefit from acute interventions.

DISCLOSURE

The author(s) declared no potential conflicts of interest with respect to the research, authorship, and/or publication of this article.

REFERENCES

1. Available at:The Top 10 causes of death. World Health Organization; 2020 https://www.who.int/news-room/fact-sheets/detail/the-top-10-causes-of-death. [Accessed 9 August 2023].
2. Aviv RI, Mandelcorn J, Chakraborty S, et al. Alberta Stroke Program Early CT Scoring of CT perfusion in early stroke visualization and assessment. AJNR Am J Neuroradiol 2007;28(10):1975–80.
3. Puetz V, Sylaja PN, Coutts SB, et al. Extent of hypoattenuation on CT angiography source images predicts functional outcome in patients with basilar artery occlusion. Stroke 2008;39(9):2485–90.
4. Tan IYL, Demchuk AM, Hopyan J, et al. CT angiography clot burden score and collateral score: Correlation with clinical and radiologic outcomes in acute middle cerebral artery infarct. Am J Neuroradiol 2009;30(3). https://doi.org/10.3174/ajnr.A1408.
5. Bae KT. Intravenous contrast medium administration and scan timing at CT: Considerations and approaches. Radiology 2010;256(1):32–61.
6. Menon BK, D'Esterre CD, Qazi EM, et al. Multiphase CT Angiography: A New Tool for the Imaging Triage of Patients with Acute Ischemic Stroke. Radiology 2015;275(2):510–20.
7. Van Rooij WJ, Peluso JPP, Sluzewski M, et al. Additional Value of 3D Rotational Angiography in Angiographically Negative Aneurysmal Subarachnoid Hemorrhage: How Negative Is Negative? AJNR Am J Neuroradiol 2008;29(5):962.
8. Hirai T, Korogi Y, Ono K, et al. Preoperative evaluation of intracranial aneurysms: usefulness of intraarterial 3D CT angiography and conventional angiography with a combined unit–initial experience. Radiology 2001;220(2):499–505.
9. Frontera JA, Claassen J, Schmidt JM, et al. Prediction of symptomatic vasospasm after subarachnoid hemorrhage: the modified fisher scale. Neurosurgery 2006;59(1):21–7.
10. Wintermark M, Flanders AE, Velthuis B, et al. Perfusion-CT assessment of infarct core and penumbra: receiver operating characteristic curve analysis in 130 patients suspected of acute hemispheric stroke. Stroke 2006;37(4):979–85.
11. Sanelli PC, Lev MH, Eastwood JD, et al. The effect of varying user-selected input parameters on quantitative values in CT perfusion maps. Acad Radiol 2004;11(10):1085–92.
12. Fieselmann A, Kowarschik M, Ganguly A, et al. Deconvolution-Based CT and MR Brain Perfusion Measurement: Theoretical Model Revisited and Practical Implementation Details. Int J Biomed Imag 2011;2011:20.
13. Kudo K, Christensen S, Sasaki M, et al. Accuracy and reliability assessment of CT and MR perfusion analysis software using a digital phantom. Radiology 2013;267(1):201–11.
14. Campbell BCV, Christensen S, Tress BM, et al. Failure of collateral blood flow is associated with infarct growth in ischemic stroke. J Cerebr Blood Flow Metabol 2013;33(8):1168–72.
15. Lansberg MG, Christensen S, Kemp S, et al. Computed tomographic perfusion to Predict

Response to Recanalization in ischemic stroke. Ann Neurol 2017;81(6):849–56.

16. Vergouwen MDI, Etminan N, Ilodigwe D, et al. Lower incidence of cerebral infarction correlates with improved functional outcome after aneurysmal subarachnoid hemorrhage. J Cerebr Blood Flow Metabol 2011;31(7):1545–53.

17. Millikan CH. Cerebral Vasospasm and Ruptured Intracranial Aneurysm. Arch Neurol 1975;32(7):433–49.

18. Taran S, Mandell DM, McCredie VA. CT Perfusion for the Detection of Delayed Cerebral Ischemia in the Presence of Neurologic Confounders. Neurocritical Care 2020;33(1):317–22.

19. Lin L, Bivard A, Parsons MW. Perfusion Patterns of Ischemic Stroke on Computed Tomography Perfusion. J Stroke 2013;15(3):164.

20. Wintermark M, Albers GW, Broderick JP, et al. Acute stroke imaging research roadmap II. Stroke 2013; 44(9):2628–39.

21. Perazella MA. Current status of gadolinium toxicity in patients with kidney disease. Clin J Am Soc Nephrol 2009;4(2):461–9.

22. Brenner DJ, Hall EJ. Computed tomography–an increasing source of radiation exposure. N Engl J Med 2007;357(22):2277–84.

23. Othman AE, Afat S, Nikoubashman O, et al. Volume perfusion CT imaging of cerebral vasospasm: diagnostic performance of different perfusion maps. Neuroradiology 2016;58(8):787–92.

24. Souza LCS, Yoo AJ, Chaudhry ZA, et al. Malignant CTA collateral profile is highly specific for large admission DWI infarct core and poor outcome in acute stroke. AJNR Am J Neuroradiol 2012;33(7): 1331–6.

25. Hoeffner EG, Case I, Jain R, et al. Cerebral perfusion CT: technique and clinical applications. Radiology 2004;231(3):632–44.

26. Hacke W, Albers G, Al-Rawi Y, et al. The Desmoteplase in Acute Ischemic Stroke Trial (DIAS): a phase II MRI-based 9-hour window acute stroke thrombolysis trial with intravenous desmoteplase. Stroke 2005;36(1):66–73.

27. Albers GW, Marks MP, Kemp S, et al. Thrombectomy for Stroke at 6 to 16 Hours with Selection by Perfusion Imaging. N Engl J Med 2018;378(8):708–18.

28. Nogueira RG, Jadhav AP, Haussen DC, et al. Thrombectomy 6 to 24 Hours after Stroke with a Mismatch between Deficit and Infarct. N Engl J Med 2018; 378(1):11–21.

29. Dani KA, Thomas RGR, Chappell FM, et al. Computed tomography and magnetic resonance perfusion imaging in ischemic stroke: definitions and thresholds. Ann Neurol 2011;70(3):384–401.

Transcranial Ultrasound in the Neurocritical Care Unit

Venkatakrishna Rajajee, MBBS

KEYWORDS

- Ultrasonography • Transcranial Doppler ultrasonography • Cerebral vasospasm
- Intracranial pressure

KEY POINTS

- Traditional nonimaging transcranial Doppler (TCD) permits evaluation of cerebral blood flow velocities within large intracranial arteries, whereas transcranial color-coded sonography additionally allows B-mode imaging of parenchyma and duplex evaluation.
- Time-averaged peak velocities (TAPVs) in the middle cerebral artery >120 cm/s and a Lindegaard ratio >3 indicate the presence of cerebral vasospasm, whereas TAPVs > 200 cm/s and a Lindegaard ratio >6 indicate severe vasospasm.
- The TCD pulsatility index and Czosnyka formula have a high negative predictive value for the identification of elevated intracranial pressure.
- The presence of short systolic spikes or oscillating flow on TCD in the bilateral anterior and posterior circulation may be used in the determination brain death.
- Transcranial B-mode imaging may be used to measure midline shift or detect ventriculomegaly.

INTRODUCTION

Transcranial ultrasound has been in use in the neurocritical care unit (NCCU) for approximately 40 years, since Rune Aaslid described the use of transcranial Doppler (TCD) to evaluate basal intracranial arteries in 1982.[1] Although the skull is a barrier to the passage of sound waves, ultrasound evaluation of the brain is possible through several "windows"—large foramina or skull regions with relatively thin bone. Although limited B-mode imaging of the brain is feasible and has potential clinical applications, the primary focus of transcranial ultrasound has been the Doppler evaluation of large intracranial arteries. In this article, the clinical applications of transcranial ultrasound in critically ill patients will be reviewed. The use of TCD to measure cerebral blood flow velocity (CBFV) has been the primary bedside technique used to monitor patients with aneurysmal subarachnoid hemorrhage (aSAH) for the development of large vessel vasospasm (LVV), following the original description by Aaslid in 1984.[2] TCD may also be used to estimate cerebral perfusion pressure (CPP) and evaluate intracranial pressure (ICP). Blood flow is profoundly impaired as patients with devastating brain injury progress to brain death, and TCD may be used as a confirmatory test for the determination of death by neurologic criteria. Although several other cerebrovascular applications exist, such as the assessment of recanalization following acute ischemic stroke, evaluation for intracranial stenosis, screening for chronic transfusion therapy in sickle cell disease, monitoring for cerebral emboli and assessment of cerebrovascular autoregulation, they are beyond the scope of this article, because their use in the NCCU is limited.

EQUIPMENT

Traditional TCD evaluation has been performed with specialized equipment that permits spectral Doppler evaluation. A low-frequency (2–3.5 MHz) transducer is applied to an acoustic window. Intracranial arteries are located with careful

Departments of Neurosurgery & Neurology, University of Michigan, 3552 Taubman Health Care Center, SPC 5338 1500 East Medical Center Drive, Ann Arbor, MI 48109, USA
E-mail address: venkatak@med.umich.edu

neuroimaging.theclinics.com

Neuroimag Clin N Am 34 (2024) 191–202
https://doi.org/10.1016/j.nic.2023.11.001
1052-5149/24/© 2023 Elsevier Inc. All rights reserved.

Table 1
Transcranial Doppler: Vessel characteristics

Vessel	Window	Depth (mm)	Direction of Flow Relative to Transducer	Velocity Range (cm/s)
Middle cerebral artery M2 segment	Transtemporal	30–40	Mostly toward, may curve away	30–80
Middle cerebral artery M1 segment	Transtemporal	40–65	Toward	30–80
Anterior cerebral artery A1 segment	Transtemporal	60–75	Away	30–80
Posterior cerebral artery P1 segment	Transtemporal	55–75	Toward	20–60
Posterior cerebral artery P2 segment	Transtemporal	55–75	Away	20–60
Basilar artery	Transforaminal	80–105	Away	20–60
Vertebral artery	Transforaminal	40–75	Away	20–50
Extracranial internal carotid artery	Submandibular	40–60	Away	20–50
Ophthalmic artery	Transorbital	40–50	Toward	Variable
Internal carotid artery siphon	Transorbital	58–65	Toward and away	20–70

manipulation, with changes in the depth of the pulsed wave Doppler (PWD) sample volume. Typical depths of major intracranial arteries are listed in Table 1. Power motion-mode Doppler is an innovation of nonimaging TCD that permits simultaneous PWD assessment of a more extensive linear region of brain.[3] As originally described, this was accomplished with 33 sample volumes with 2 mm spacing.[3] In addition to depiction of Doppler signal intensity and direction (red for flow toward the probe, blue for flow away) in all of these sampled regions in an M-mode format, a spectrogram is displayed from a user-selected region.

Transcranial color-coded sonography (TCCS), which this article focuses on, is typically performed with multipurpose ultrasound machines, including point-of-care ultrasound (POCUS) machines widely available in most intensive care units (ICUs). It is therefore more widely accessible, although transcranial preset software is required for POCUS machines. A low-frequency (1–5 MHz) phased-array transducer with a relatively small footprint—often the same probe used for echocardiography—is used. TCCS, which permits B-mode imaging and duplex evaluation, with visualization of the major basal intracranial arteries, offers several advantages over nonimaging TCD. Duplex imaging permits optimization of, and correction for, the angle of insonation and therefore more accurate measurement of velocity. In contrast, the angle of insonation with nonimaging TCD frequently exceeds 30° to 60°, which leads to significant underestimation of CBFV.[4–6] Localization of vessels—and identification of vessel segments of interest—is easier with TCCS than with traditional TCD, especially for inexperienced operators. B-mode imaging of brain parenchyma may have additional clinical utility. The disadvantages of TCCS include a larger transducer footprint, which may complicate insonation through small acoustic windows, and the relative insensitivity of duplex imaging to vessels with low flow. In addition, while correction of velocities for angle of insonation with TCCS yields more technically accurate velocities, the best validated diagnostic thresholds for conditions such as cerebral vasospasm have been established using traditional TCD, without angle correction.

IMAGING TECHNIQUE AND NORMAL ANATOMY WITH TRANSCRANIAL COLOR-CODED SONOGRAPHY

The *transtemporal* acoustic window permits interrogation of the large arteries at the base of the brain. The transducer is positioned above the zygomatic arch, immediately anterior to the upper pinna (Fig. 1). The index mark on the transducer should point anteriorly and superiorly, at a 10° to 20° angle to the axial plane with the transducer tilted and pointing slightly cephalad, also at a 10°

to 20° angle cephalad to the axial plane. If no recognizable anatomic features are visible despite adjustment of probe position, it is possible the patient does not have an adequate acoustic window. The most recognizable structure is the midbrain, with the "mickey mouse ears" of the crus cerebri (Fig. 2). Further cephalad angulation of the transducer reveals the third, followed by the lateral, ventricles. In the absence of ventriculomegaly, the third and lateral ventricles may only be identified by the presence of hyperechoic choroid plexus (Fig. 3). Duplex examination is then performed in the mesencephalic plane, with the color box positioned over the expected location of major intracranial arteries within the basal cisterns (Fig. 4). The middle cerebral artery (MCA), depicted in red by convention with blood flow toward the transducer, courses through the sylvian fissure to bifurcate into the M2 superior and inferior divisions. The anterior cerebral artery (ACA) A1 segment (depicted in blue, with flow away from the transducer) is seen extending anteriorly and toward the midline from the internal carotid artery (ICA) bifurcation, where it meets the contralateral A1 segment (depicted in red, with flow toward the transducer). The A2 segments typically cannot be individually distinguished or interrogated with spectral Doppler because of a nearly 90° angle of insonation. A slight caudal tilt of the transducer will reveal the intracranial ICA proximal to the bifurcation. The posterior cerebral artery (PCA) is visible curving around the crus cerebri, with the P1 segment in red and the P2 segment in blue. The posterior communicating artery (PComm) artery is often visible, connecting the distal ICA to

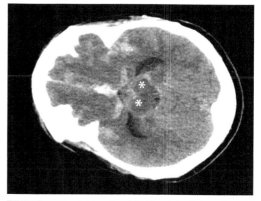

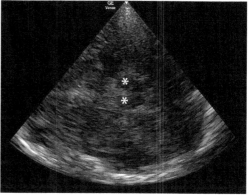

Fig. 2. Comparison of CT (*top*) and transtemporal B-mode ultrasound (*bottom*) images at the mesencephalic level. * represents the crus cerebri.

the PCA. Contralateral vessels are often visible when depth is increased to 13 cm or greater, with directions of flow reversed compared to the ipsilateral side (see Fig. 4).

The *transforaminal* window, through the foramen magnum, permits evaluation of the vertebrobasilar circulation. The patient's head is flexed forward and the transducer positioned in the suboccipital

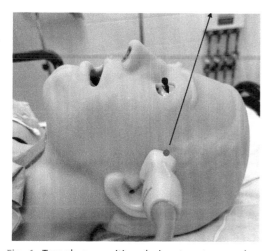

Fig. 1. Transducer position during transtemporal sonography. The red dot and black arrow represent the angle and direction of the index mark on the transducer.

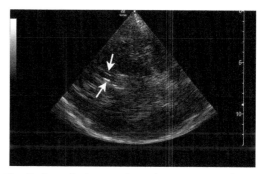

Fig. 3. B-mode image through transtemporal window, superior to the mesencephalic plane. White arrows point to hyperechoic choroid plexus within the lateral ventricles on either side.

A

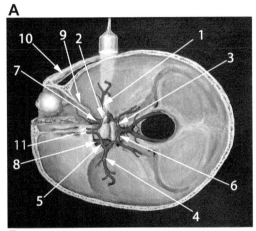

B

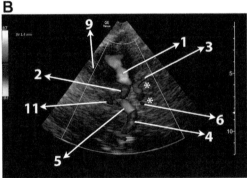

Fig. 4. Transtemporal Doppler evaluation of basal intracranial arteries-pictorial depiction (A) and duplex imaging (B). 1, Ipsilateral middle cerebral artery (MCA); 2, ipsilateral anterior cerebral artery (ACA); 3, ipsilateral posterior cerebral artery (PCA); 4, contralateral MCA; 5, contralateral ACA; 6, contralateral PCA; 7, ipsilateral intracranial ICA; 8, contralateral intracranial ICA; 9, ipsilateral greater wing of the sphenoid bone; 10, ipsilateral zygomatic arch; 11, bilateral anterior cerebral artery A2 segments. (Pictorial depiction is *adapted from* an open-source image by Rune Aaslid (https://transcranial.com/).

region, pointing toward the nasion, with the index mark pointing to the right. The foramen magnum is visible as a circular hypoechoic structure. Positioning the color box over the foramen magnum reveals the V4 segments of the vertebral arteries on either side (Fig. 5). Beyond the confluence, the basilar artery is seen extending intracranially.

The *submandibular* window permits evaluation of the distal, cervical, extracranial ICA (exICA). The transducer is positioned in the submandibular region, pointing superiorly, medially, and slightly posteriorly. The exICA is visible on duplex as a linear structure in blue medial to the internal jugular vein (Fig. 6). The *transorbital* window, with insonation through the orbit, allows visualization of the carotid siphon and the ophthalmic artery but is of limited value in the ICU.

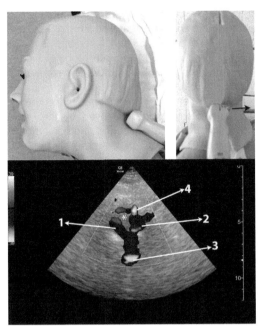

Fig. 5. Transforaminal window. Transducer position (*top*) (red index mark on the transducer points to patient's right) and duplex image (*bottom*). * indicates foramen magnum. 1, right vertebral artery; 2, left vertebral artery; 3, basilar artery; 4, left posterior inferior cerebellar artery origin.

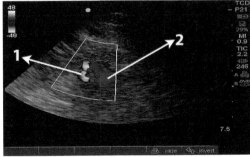

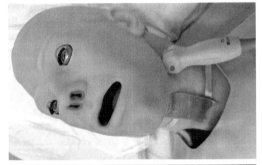

Fig. 6. Submandibular insonation. Transducer position (*top*) (red index mark on transducer points anteriorly and medially). Duplex image (*bottom*). 1, distal extracranial internal carotid artery; 2, internal jugular vein.

Following identification of the major intracranial arteries, PWD evaluation is performed. A 3 to 10 mm sample volume is positioned on the arterial segment of interest and the spectral waveform obtained (Fig. 7). The angle of insonation should ideally be less than 30°, achieved through the selection of an appropriate location on the artery and slight modifications of transducer position within the acoustic window. Velocities should not be measured with an angle of insonation greater than 60°. The angle of insonation can be measured with a direction-of-flow indicator and measured velocities corrected for angle of insonation (see Fig. 7). The waveform through a single cardiac cycle is traced, yielding the peak systolic velocity (PSV), end-diastolic velocity (EDV) and time-averaged peak velocity (TAPV), often referred to as "mean" CBFV. The Gosling pulsatility index (PI) is calculated as (PSV-EDV)/TAPV and is automatically displayed on most machines.

CLINICAL APPLICATIONS
Cerebral Vasospasm Following Subarachnoid Hemorrhage

Some degree of LVV is common following aSAH, although most patients with LVV remain asymptomatic through their hospital course. Approximately 30% of aSAH patients will suffer neurologic deterioration and/or the appearance of new infarcts on imaging caused by delayed cerebral ischemia (DCI).[7,8] Unlike LVV, DCI is independently associated with poor long-term functional outcome.[8] Although DCI is multifactorial,[9] and a likely consequence of the inflammatory response to aSAH, LVV and DCI are closely related. Several studies suggest that LVV is a strong independent predictor of DCI.[10,11] Therefore, although the goal of serial TCD examination is to identify SAH patients at high risk for DCI, this is primarily achieved through the detection of LVV. In addition, TCD examination of aSAH patients who suffer neurologic deterioration can help identify DCI as the likely etiology, facilitating urgent treatment. Vasospasm is identified through the elevation in CBFV that occurs as luminal diameter decreases.

$$\text{Flow} = \text{Velocity} \times \text{Area} (\pi r^2)$$

Therefore, $\text{Velocity} = \text{Flow}/\pi r^2$

Velocity is inversely proportional to the square of the radius, leading to a measurable increase in CBFV with increasing vasospasm. However, an increase in velocity may also occur through increased flow. A hyperdynamic circulation that increases flow is common in patients with aSAH, as a consequence of sympathetic activation.[12]

Diagnostic Criteria

The best validated criteria for the diagnosis of LVV were edtablished using traditional "blind" TCD and interrogation of the MCA. A TAPV greater than 120 cm/s in the MCA is most widely used for the diagnosis of vasospasm, whereas a TAPV greater than 200 cm/s represents severe vasospasm, often defined as greater than 50% narrowing of luminal diameter.[7,13,14] A ratio of intracranial to

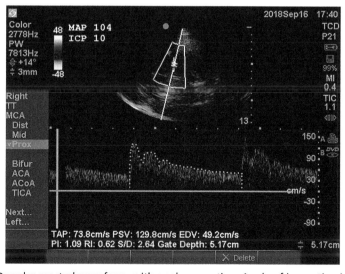

Fig. 7. Transcranial Doppler spectral waveform, with angle correction. Angle of insonation is 14°. Time-averaged peak velocity (TAP) is 73.8 cm/s, peak systolic velocity (PSV) is 129.8 cm/s, end-diastolic velocity (EDV) 49.2 cm/s, pulsatility index (PI) is 1.09, mean arterial pressure (MAP) is 104 mm Hg, and intracranial pressure (ICP) measured from the invasive monitor is 10 mm Hg. Estimated ICP using the Czosnyka formula is calculated at 21 mm Hg, which overestimates the actual ICP.

extracranial flow velocity is often used to distinguish the contribution of vasospasm and hyperdynamic circulation to elevated MCA TAPV. The Lindegaard ratio is the ratio of TAPV measured in the MCA M1 segment to the TAPV measured in the terminal exICA.[14] Of note, measurement of exICA TAPV should be performed through a submandibular window with a phased array transducer and TCD software, rather than a linear transducer with carotid Doppler software, which will instead yield a mean velocity. The Lindegaard ratio is primarily of value with an elevated MCA TAPV. In this setting, a ratio less than 3 represents hyperdynamic flow, 3 to 6 represents mild to moderate vasospasm, and greater than 6 represents severe vasospasm.[14] Although a similar elevation in velocity in any other large artery likely represents the presence of LVV, there has been insufficient validation of diagnostic thresholds in other vessels. A ratio of basilar artery velocity to average *extracranial* vertebral artery velocity greater than 2 may be used to identify LVV,[15] whereas a ratio greater than 3 may represent greater than 50% luminal narrowing of the basilar artery.[16] Although angle-corrected velocities more accurately represent "true" CBFV, they are higher than velocities measured without angle correction.[6,17,18] Although limited work has been performed to validate angle-corrected velocities for the diagnosis of LVV, these are not yet in widespread use in clinical practice.[17,19] Arterial segments in spasm may be visually identified through the presence of aliasing on TCCS duplex imaging (Fig. 8). The color velocity scale should be sufficiently high, because a low pulse repetition frequency will result in aliasing at relatively normal velocities.

Although elevated velocities may indicate LVV, they do not provide information on perfusion of cerebral tissue. The PI may provide additional information on perfusion status, because the cerebral autoregulatory response to hypoperfusion caused by a severely stenotic vessel is vasodilation at an arteriolar level, with lower resistance to flow and a decrease in the PI. Therefore, a combination of elevated TAPV in the MCA M1 segment with low PI may represent hypoperfusion caused by vasospasm. In one study, although a TAPV greater than 140 cm/s was the optimal cutoff to predict LVV, a PI less than 0.58 best predicted DCI.[20] Of note, vasospasm that predominantly involves arterial segments distal to the point of insonation will result in increased resistance to flow and an elevation in PI.

Differential Diagnosis and Potential Pitfalls

The Lindegaard ratio is most commonly used to distinguish the contribution of hyperdynamic flow and vasospasm, as described above. Erroneous measurement of exICA TAPV, with insufficient attention to angle of insonation particularly in the presence of vessel tortuosity, may result in a steep angle and artificially low exICA velocity, leading to a falsely elevated Lindegaard ratio that raises concern for vasospasm. Less commonly, stenosis of the distal exICA or post-stenotic flow distal to stenosis at the cervical ICA bifurcation may confound velocity measurement. The most common pitfalls with TCD are technical. Acoustic windows are absent on one side in about 10% to 20% of patients and on both sides in 3% to 10%.[21,22] In these cases, the bilateral intracranial circulation can sometimes be assessed from a single side (see Fig. 4). Careful visual inspection and interrogation of all major vessel segments are required, because vasospasm may be severe in one segment and mild in an adjoining segment. As previously described, an excessive angle of insonation can lead to inaccurately low CBFV measurements. Distal segments of large arteries cannot be directly assessed with TCD, and the presence of vasospasm in these segments may only manifest as an increase in the PI measured in proximal segments. Finally, up to 20% to 30% of patients with DCI do not demonstrate LVV.[23]

CASE STUDY

A 47-year-old right-handed woman is admitted to the NCCU with aSAH from a left PComm aneurysm. She undergoes endovascular coil embolization with the placement of an external ventricular drain. She is alert and fully oriented. She undergoes daily bedside TCD evaluation. Day 2 velocities in all intracranial arteries evaluated are less than 100 cm/s and PIs are 0.8 to 1.2. Four days following aneurysm rupture, the patient is asymptomatic. The left MCA TAPV is 170 cm/s (PI 0.82) and right MCA TAPV is 156 cm/s (PI 0.9). Left exICA TAPV is 40 cm/s and the right exICA TAPV is 42 cm/s. On day 10, she is noticed to have mild word finding difficulty and worsening confusion, along with a minimal right-sided pronator drift. Urgent POCUS-TCCS evaluation reveals severe aliasing in multiple vessels. Left MCA TAPV is 253 cm/s (PI 0.34), right MCA TAPV 203 cm/s (PI 0.55), left exICA TAPV 38 cm/s, and right exICA TAPV 40 cm/s.

Interpretation and management: Initial TCD evaluation and the clinical examination were reassuring. Evaluation on day 4 revealed some increase in velocities; however, the Lindegaard ratios were 4.25 on the left and 3.71 on the right, suggesting relatively mild LVV. This alerts the clinician to the potential to develop DCI. In this

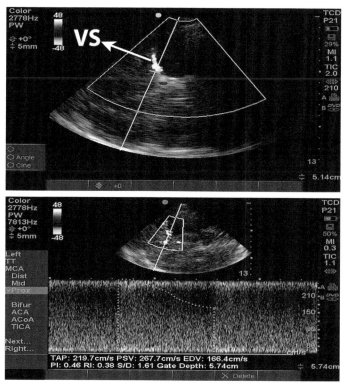

Fig. 8. Severe cerebral vasospasm. Duplex image (*top*) demonstrates aliasing (bright blue region within the otherwise red/orange/yellow M1 segment of the left middle cerebral artery, VS = vasospasm). Whereas aliasing may simply reflect the limits of the color scale, pulse Doppler evaluation (*bottom*) demonstrates a time averaged peak (TAP) > 219 cm/s within the region of aliasing, suggesting severe vasospasm.

context, the relatively mild symptoms noticed on day 10 trigger an immediate and proactive response by the clinical team. Repeat TCD evaluation reveals a Lindegaard ratio of 6.66 on the left and 5.07 on the right, suggesting severe vasospasm on the left and at least moderate vasospasm on the right. Most concerning, the corresponding PIs are low, particularly on the left, suggesting an attempt by the patient's preserved autoregulation to compensate for tissue hypoperfusion. The symptoms and TCD findings are consistent with DCI. A norepinephrine infusion is titrated to achieve a 30% increase in the mean arterial pressure (MAP), to improve perfusion of ischemic regions of the brain.[24,25] Computed tomography (CT) angiography confirms the presence of diffuse LVV, with especially severe vasospasm in the left anterior circulation. CT perfusion reveals a 23 mL region of hypoperfusion (Tmax >6 seconds) in the left ACA–MCA borderzone territory, with no core infarct. Three hours following hemodynamic augmentation, she is again neurologically intact. Hemodynamic augmentation is slowly weaned off over several days. She is independent to activities of daily living at her 6-month clinic visit.

Elevated Intracranial Pressure

Patients with severe brain injury are at risk for elevated ICP, cerebral herniation, and death. Although invasive ICP monitoring is the gold standard, the risk of an invasive intracranial procedure may be unacceptably high in coagulopathic patients, such as those with acute liver failure (ALF). In addition, resource-constrained environments, such as those in low- and middle-income countries, remote rural regions and tactical combat military care locations may lack the necessary resources. POCUS may have value in these situations to screen patients for the presence of life-threatening ICP elevation.

Although many different TCD techniques have been studied for the assessment of ICP,[26] this article focuses on two techniques that can be performed with widely available ultrasound machines. The first is the PI, which increases as elevated ICP increases resistance to flow. Although a normal PI may suggest a severe elevation in ICP is unlikely, the specificity of an elevated PI is poor because multiple factors can elevate distal resistance. This includes small vessel disease, autoregulatory vasoconstriction, and distal vessel stenosis or spasm. It is also possible to estimate CPP with TCD. Czosnyka and colleagues described estimation of CPP (CPPe) in 96 patients with traumatic brain injury (TBI).[27] The assessment of MCA-CBFV was performed using a continuous TCD band for 20 to 120 minutes, with concomitant MAP and invasive ICP monitoring. Continuous ICP, MAP, and TCD-CBFV data for the 20 to 120 minutes were converted from digital to analog signal, with time integration of waveform signals for 5-s periods. Spectral filtration was used to minimize artifact and Fourier transformation performed to evaluate the first harmonic components of the arterial (A1) and CBFV (F1) waveforms. CPPe was calculated using the formula:

CPPe = [MAP × (CBFV-diastolic / CBFV-mean)] + 14

Estimated ICP (ICPe) = MAP − CPPe.

The number 14 was a specific correction factor for TBI. In this study, correlation of CPP and CPPe was good ($r = 0.73$), with estimation error less than 10 mm Hg in 71% examinations and positive predictive power 94% for the detection of CPP less than 60 mm Hg. Subsequent studies have demonstrated variable results.[27–32,42] A recent international multicenter study of diagnostic accuracy (IMPRESSIT-2) demonstrated an area under the curve 0.76 and negative predictive value (NPV) 96% for detection of ICP greater than 22 mm Hg.[31]

Diagnostic Criteria

In a recent study, an ICPe greater than 21 mm Hg had an NPV 100% for ICP greater than 22 mm Hg, when assessment was performed with TCCS and angle correction (see Fig. 7).[42] We use this threshold, along with a PI less than 0.82, which also demonstrated an NPV of 100% in the same study, to identify patients unlikely to have elevated ICP at the time of evaluation. Specificity is, however, poor: 30% for ICPe greater than 21 mm Hg and a PI greater than 0.82.[42]

Differential Diagnosis and Potential Pitfalls

A variety of factors can result in false-positive elevation in the ICPe and PI. This includes focal unilateral or multifocal bilateral pathology (such as ischemic stroke) in the MCA distribution, small vessel disease, multifocal distal vasospasm/stenosis, and autoregulatory arteriolar vasoconstriction.

The assessment of ICP with TCD is not continuous. The general limitations of TCD, such as an absent acoustic window and the importance of insonation angle, have been discussed. In one study, the use of TCCS to perform angle correction greatly increased the accuracy of ICP estimation with TCD.[42] It should also be noted that the original validation of this technique was performed with continuous TCD and time integration of measurements, with spectral filtration to minimize noise and Fourier transformation of waveforms.[27] This requires specialized equipment, compared with the point-in-time assessments actually performed at most centers while evaluating ICP with this technique. All validation studies have demonstrated relatively broad confidence intervals for accuracy. TCD should therefore not be used in isolation to guide ICP management and should be integrated with other data, such as CT imaging and pupillometry.[32]

CASE STUDY

A 23-year-old woman suffers rapid deterioration in mental status and requires intubation 4 days following admission for an acetaminophen overdose. The Glasgow coma scale is 3, bilateral pupils are reactive. Non-contrast CT demonstrates mild diffuse sulcal effacement consistent with cerebral edema caused by ALF. The international normalized ratio is 4.0, and invasive ICP monitor placement is considered unacceptably risky by the consulting neurosurgeon. TCD evaluation reveals an ICPe 14 mm Hg and PI of 0.68 (average of both sides for both measures), reassuring for normal ICP despite the poor neurologic examination. She undergoes liver transplantation and regains consciousness over several days. She is neurologically intact 6 months following the initial admission.

Brain Death Evaluation

Progressive and uncontrolled elevation in ICP in the setting of devastating brain injury will eventually result in ICP that exceeds perfusion pressure. The brain is critically dependent on continuous forward flow through the cardiac cycle, including in diastole. However, as brain death approaches and ICP exceeds diastolic blood pressure, TCD evaluation will demonstrate purely systolic flow. Eventually, only *short systolic spikes* in flow are recorded (Fig. 9). Some large vessels such as the MCA may demonstrate *reverberating (oscillating) flow* in nearly stagnant columns of blood, with short systolic spikes and retrograde diastolic flow (Fig. 10). These waveforms are incompatible with life, unless the underlying condition is rapidly reversed. In conjunction with clinical evidence of

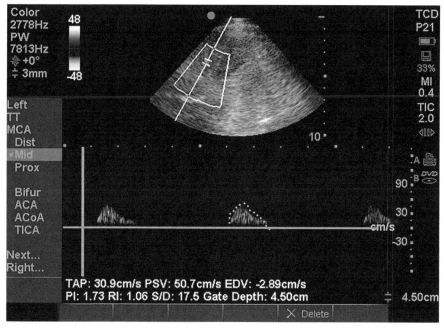

Fig. 9. Short systolic spikes. Pulse Doppler evaluation of the middle cerebral artery reveals only short systolic spikes in antegrade flow, with absent diastolic flow. The patient subsequently met criteria for brain death.

loss of brainstem function, TCD may therefore be used as a confirmatory test for brain death.[33,34]

Diagnostic Criteria

The World Brain Death Project suggests the following criteria for the use of TCD as a confirmatory test for the determination of death by neurologic criteria in adults.[34]

1. Two examinations at least 30 minutes apart.

2. Evaluate the bilateral anterior and posterior circulation, to include both ICAs and the vertebrobasilar circulation.

3. The examinations must illustrate biphasic oscillating flow and systolic spikes with reversal of flow in diastole.

Differential Diagnosis and Potential Pitfalls

Given the absence of acoustic windows in 10% to 20% of patients, the inability to detect flow within

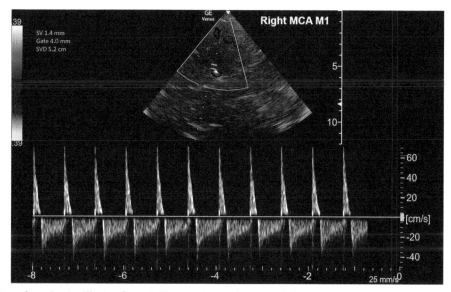

Fig. 10. Reverberating/oscillating flow. Pulse Doppler evaluation of the middle cerebral artery reveals only systolic spikes in antegrade flow, followed by retrograde flow. The patient subsequently met criteria for brain death.

intracranial vessels alone should *not* be used for the determination of death by neurologic criteria-oscillating flow or short systolic spikes should be demonstrated. These waveforms may, however, be seen unilaterally, with focal pathology, such a large ischemic stroke. It is critical therefore that these waveforms be recorded in *both* MCA/ICAs and the basilar artery. In the setting of rapidly progressive but reversible intracranial pathology such as an expanding acute subdural hematoma or hydrocephalus, the focus must be on management: reversal of cerebral herniation and surgical decompression. TCD evaluation in this setting may reveal profound alterations concerning for cerebral circulatory arrest; however, in the hyperacute setting, urgent treatment and reversal of pathology may result in restoration of flow and neurologic recovery.[35]

Transcranial B-Mode Imaging

Although visualization of anatomic detail with B-mode imaging is possible in the presence of a craniectomy defect (or a fontanelle in a child), delineation of anatomy through transtemporal windows is typically poor. The normal ventricular system may only be visible through the presence of hyperechoic choroid plexus (see Fig. 3). In the presence of hydrocephalus, however, the hypoechoic ventricles may be clearly visible. The assessment of ventriculomegaly with transcranial ultrasound has been reported to compare favorably to CT assessment.[36,37] Transtemporal B-mode ultrasound may also be used to measure midline shift. The distance from the transducer to the hyperechoic choroid plexus in the third ventricle is measured on each side. Midline shift is then calculated as half the difference between these two measurements (Fig. 11).[38,39] Preliminary studies also suggest that intraparenchymal hematomas may be detected and measured with transcranial B-mode ultrasound.[40–42] Although promising, given the widespread availability of CT, transcranial B-mode imaging has seen limited use in clinical practice.

SUMMARY

Although TCD has long been used to monitor patients with SAH for cerebral vasospasm, TCCS may also be used to assess the risk of DCI, screen patients for the presence of elevated ICP, confirm the diagnosis of brain death, measure midline shift, and detect ventriculomegaly. TCCS should therefore be integrated with other POCUS techniques as an essential skill for the neurointensivist.

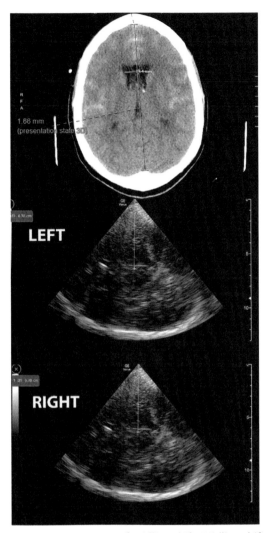

Fig. 11. Measurement of midline shift. Midline shift 1.6 mm measured from CT (*top*). The transtemporal B-mode image on the left reveals a distance of 6.59 cm (*A*) from transducer to the third ventricle (*middle*). The corresponding distance on the right (*bottom*) is 6.38 cm (*B*). Midline shift = (A - B)/ 2 = 1.05 mm.

DISCLOSURE

Dr Rajajee has received funding from the National Institutes of Health, United States and Department of Defense, United States to study optic nerve ultrasound and transcranial Doppler as noninvasive intracranial pressure assessment tools.

REFERENCES

1. Aaslid R, Markwalder TM, Nornes H. Noninvasive transcranial Doppler ultrasound recording of flow velocity in basal cerebral arteries. J Neurosurg 1982;57(6):769–74.

2. Aaslid R, Huber P, Nornes H. Evaluation of cerebro-vascular spasm with transcranial Doppler ultrasound. J Neurosurg 1984;60(1):37–41.

3. Moehring MA, Spencer MP. Power M-mode Doppler (PMD) for observing cerebral blood flow and tracking emboli. Ultrasound Med Biol 2002;28(1):49–57.

4. Krejza J, Mariak Z, Babikian VL. Importance of angle correction in the measurement of blood flow velocity with transcranial Doppler sonography. AJNR Am J Neuroradiol 2001;22(9):1743–7.

5. Lepic T, Veljancic D, Jovanikic O, et al. Importance of angle correction in transcranial color-coded duplex insonation of arteries at the base of the brain. Vojnosanit Pregl 2015;72(12):1093–7.

6. Schoning M, Buchholz R, Walter J. Comparative study of transcranial color duplex sonography and transcranial Doppler sonography in adults. J Neurosurg 1993;78(5):776–84.

7. Hoh BL, Ko NU, Amin-Hanjani S, et al. 2023 Guideline for the management of patients with aneurysmal subarachnoid hemorrhage: a guideline from the American Heart Association/American Stroke Association. Stroke 2023;54(7):e314–70.

8. Frontera JA, Fernandez A, Schmidt JM, et al. Defining vasospasm after subarachnoid hemorrhage: what is the most clinically relevant definition? Stroke 2009;40(6):1963–8.

9. Geraghty JR, Testai FD. Delayed cerebral ischemia after subarachnoid hemorrhage: beyond vasospasm and towards a multifactorial pathophysiology. Curr Atheroscler Rep 2017;19(12):50.

10. Crowley RW, Medel R, Dumont AS, et al. Angiographic vasospasm is strongly correlated with cerebral infarction after subarachnoid hemorrhage. Stroke 2011;42(4):919–23.

11. Nguyen AM, Williamson CA, Pandey AS, et al. Screening computed tomography angiography to identify patients at low risk for delayed cerebral ischemia following aneurysmal subarachnoid hemorrhage. Front Neurol 2021;12:740241.

12. Naredi S, Lambert G, Eden E, et al. Increased sympathetic nervous activity in patients with nontraumatic subarachnoid hemorrhage. Stroke 2000;31(4):901–6.

13. Aaslid R, Huber P, Nornes H. A transcranial Doppler method in the evaluation of cerebrovascular spasm. Neuroradiology 1986;28(1):11–6.

14. Lindegaard KF, Nornes H, Bakke SJ, et al. Cerebral vasospasm diagnosis by means of angiography and blood velocity measurements. Acta Neurochir 1989;100(1–2):12–24.

15. Soustiel JF, Shik V, Shreiber R, et al. Basilar vasospasm diagnosis: investigation of a modified "Lindegaard Index" based on imaging studies and blood velocity measurements of the basilar artery. Stroke 2002;33(1):72–7.

16. Sviri GE, Ghodke B, Britz GW, et al. Transcranial Doppler grading criteria for basilar artery vasospasm. Neurosurgery 2006;59(2):360–6. discussion 360-366.

17. Swiat M, Weigele J, Hurst RW, et al. Middle cerebral artery vasospasm: transcranial color-coded duplex sonography versus conventional nonimaging transcranial Doppler sonography. Crit Care Med 2009;37(3):963–8.

18. Rajajee V, Soroushmehr R, Williamson CA, et al. Transcranial Color-Coded Sonography With Angle Correction As a Screening Tool for Raised Intracranial Pressure. Crit Care Explor 2023;5(9):e0953.

19. Krejza J, Kochanowicz J, Mariak Z, et al. Middle cerebral artery spasm after subarachnoid hemorrhage: detection with transcranial color-coded duplex US. Radiology 2005;236(2):621–9.

20. Rajajee V, Fletcher JJ, Pandey AS, et al. Low pulsatility index on transcranial Doppler predicts symptomatic large-vessel vasospasm after aneurysmal subarachnoid hemorrhage. Neurosurgery 2012;70(5):1195–206. discussion 1206.

21. Krejza J, Swiat M, Pawlak MA, et al. Suitability of temporal bone acoustic window: conventional TCD versus transcranial color-coded duplex sonography. J Neuroimaging 2007;17(4):311–4.

22. Marinoni M, Ginanneschi A, Forleo P, et al. Technical limits in transcranial Doppler recording: inadequate acoustic windows. Ultrasound Med Biol 1997;23(8):1275–7.

23. Dhar R, Scalfani MT, Blackburn S, et al. Relationship between angiographic vasospasm and regional hypoperfusion in aneurysmal subarachnoid hemorrhage. Stroke 2012;43(7):1788–94.

24. Muench E, Horn P, Bauhuf C, et al. Effects of hypervolemia and hypertension on regional cerebral blood flow, intracranial pressure, and brain tissue oxygenation after subarachnoid hemorrhage. Crit Care Med 2007;35(8):1844–51. quiz 1852.

25. Raabe A, Beck J, Keller M, et al. Relative importance of hypertension compared with hypervolemia for increasing cerebral oxygenation in patients with cerebral vasospasm after subarachnoid hemorrhage. J Neurosurg 2005;103(6):974–81.

26. Cardim D, Robba C, Bohdanowicz M, et al. Non-invasive monitoring of intracranial pressure using transcranial Doppler ultrasonography: is it possible? Neurocritical Care 2016;25(3):473–91.

27. Czosnyka M, Matta BF, Smielewski P, et al. Cerebral perfusion pressure in head-injured patients: a noninvasive assessment using transcranial Doppler ultrasonography. J Neurosurg 1998;88(5):802–8.

28. Cardim D, Robba C, Czosnyka M, et al. Noninvasive intracranial pressure estimation with transcranial doppler: a prospective observational study. J Neurosurg Anesthesiol 2020;32(4):349–53.

29. Robba C, Cardim D, Tajsic T, et al. Ultrasound noninvasive measurement of intracranial pressure in

neurointensive care: A prospective observational study. PLoS Med 2017;14(7):e1002356.

30. Rajajee V, Williamson CA, Fontana RJ, et al. Noninvasive intracranial pressure assessment in acute liver failure. Neurocritical Care 2018;29(2):280–90.

31. Rasulo FA, Calza S, Robba C, et al. Transcranial Doppler as a screening test to exclude intracranial hypertension in brain-injured patients: the IMPRESSIT-2 prospective multicenter international study. Crit Care 2022;26(1):110.

32. Robba C, Pozzebon S, Moro B, et al. Multimodal non-invasive assessment of intracranial hypertension: an observational study. Crit Care 2020;24(1):379.

33. Monteiro LM, Bollen CW, van Huffelen AC, et al. Transcranial Doppler ultrasonography to confirm brain death: a meta-analysis. Intensive Care Med 2006;32(12):1937–44.

34. Greer DM, Shemie SD, Lewis A, et al. Determination of Brain Death/Death by Neurologic Criteria: The World Brain Death Project. JAMA 2020;324(11):1078–97.

35. Steinmetz H, Hassler W. Reversible intracranial circulatory arrest in acute subarachnoid haemorrhage. J Neurol Neurosurg Psychiatry 1988;51(10):1355–6.

36. Kiphuth IC, Huttner HB, Struffert T, et al. Sonographic monitoring of ventricle enlargement in posthemorrhagic hydrocephalus. Neurology 2011;76(10):858–62.

37. Seidel G, Kaps M, Gerriets T, et al. Evaluation of the ventricular system in adults by transcranial duplex sonography. J Neuroimaging 1995;5(2):105–8.

38. Gerriets T, Stolz E, Konig S, et al. Sonographic monitoring of midline shift in space-occupying stroke: an early outcome predictor. Stroke 2001;32(2):442–7.

39. Stolz E, Gerriets T, Fiss I, et al. Comparison of transcranial color-coded duplex sonography and cranial CT measurements for determining third ventricle midline shift in space-occupying stroke. AJNR Am J Neuroradiol 1999;20(8):1567–71.

40. Gomez-de Frutos MC, Garcia-Suarez I, Laso-Garcia F, et al. B-Mode Ultrasound, a Reliable Tool for Monitoring Experimental Intracerebral Hemorrhage. Front Neurol 2021;12:771402.

41. Maurer M, Shambal S, Berg D, et al. Differentiation between intracerebral hemorrhage and ischemic stroke by transcranial color-coded duplex-sonography. Stroke 1998;29(12):2563–7.

42. Sarwal A, Patel Y, D'Agostino R, et al. Exploratory study to assess feasibility of intracerebral hemorrhage detection by point of care cranial ultrasound. Ultrasound J 2022;14(1):40.

MR Imaging Techniques for Acute Ischemic Stroke and Delayed Cerebral Ischemia Following Subarachnoid Hemorrhage

Marco Colasurdo, MD[a,b], Huanwen Chen, MD[a,c,d],
Dheeraj Gandhi, MBBS[a,e,f],*

KEYWORDS

- Acute ischemic stroke • Advanced MR imaging • Delayed cerebral ischemia
- Subarachnoid hemorrhage

KEY POINTS

- We provide an overview of the use of MR imaging techniques to identify, characterize, and quantify important aspects of acute ischemic stroke (AIS) and delayed cerebral ischemia (DCI).
- We summarize commonly used MR sequences for AIS and DCI and highlight their clinical applications.
- We also discuss some promising investigational uses of MR imaging for AIS and DCI.

INTRODUCTION

Acute ischemic stroke (AIS) is a leading cause of death and disability worldwide, and its prevalence is expected to increase with global population aging and the burgeoning obesity epidemic.[1] Clinical care for AIS has evolved during the past 3 decades, and it comprises of 3 major tenants: (1) timely recanalization of occluded vessels with intravenous thrombolysis (IVT) or endovascular thrombectomy (EVT), (2) prompt initiation of antithrombotic agents to prevent stroke recurrences, and (3) poststroke supportive care and rehabilitation.[2] Optimal patient selection and treatment decisions for acute recanalization and secondary stroke prevention rely on thorough evaluation of patients' clinical history, neurologic examination, and multimodality neuroimaging.

Delayed cerebral ischemia (DCI) following subarachnoid hemorrhage (SAH) is another ischemic neurovascular phenomenon that portends poor neurologic outcomes, and it has emerged as an important treatment target to reduce the morbidity and mortality associated with SAH.[3] Similar to AIS, the diagnosis and treatment of DCI rely heavily on multimodality neuroimaging as well.

In this article, we provide an overview of the use of MR imaging techniques to identify, characterize, and quantify important aspects of AIS and DCI. We

[a] Division of Interventional Neuroradiology, Department of Diagnostic Radiology, University of Maryland School of Medicine, 22 South Green Street, Baltimore, MD 21201, USA; [b] Department of Interventional Radiology, Oregon Health and Science University, 3181 SW Sam Jackson Park Road, Portland, OR 97239, USA; [c] National Institute for Neurological Disorders and Stroke, National Institutes of Health, 10 center drive, Bethesda, MD 20892, USA; [d] Department of Neurology, MedStar Georgetown University Hospital, Washington, DC 20007, USA; [e] Department of Neurology, University of Maryland School of Medicine, 22 South Green Street, Baltimore, MD 21201, USA; [f] Department of Neurosurgery, University of Maryland School of Medicine, 22 South Green Street, Baltimore, MD 21201, USA
* Corresponding author. Division of Interventional Neuroradiology, Department of Diagnostic Radiology, University of Maryland School of Medicine, 22 South Green Street, Baltimore, MD 21201.
E-mail address: dgandhi@umm.edu

Neuroimag Clin N Am 34 (2024) 203–214
https://doi.org/10.1016/j.nic.2023.12.002
1052-5149/24/© 2024 Elsevier Inc. All rights reserved.

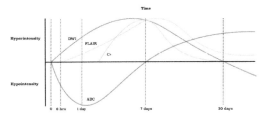

Fig. 1. Time course of MR imaging signal abnormalities for various sequences. ADC, apparent diffusion coefficient; C+, contrast enhancement; DWI, diffusion-weighted imaging; FLAIR, fluid attenuated inversion recovery.

summarize commonly used MR sequences for AIS and DCI and highlight their clinical applications. We also discuss some promising investigational uses of MR imaging for AIS and DCI.

MR IMAGING FOR TISSUE CHARACTERIZATION IN ACUTE ISCHEMIC STROKE

To understand MR imaging for acute ischemic strokes, one must first appreciate their underlying pathophysiology. The first consequence of brain tissue ischemia is the failure of Na^+/K^+ ATPase pumps on the cell surfaces, which leads to intracellular retention of sodium and thus creating a net influx of free water and cytotoxic edema.[4] As ischemic conditions persist, rupture and death of ischemic cells releases intracellular contents into the interstitial space, thereby increasing the osmolality of the interstitial space, leading to vasogenic edema.[5] Prolonged ischemia can also cause disruptions in the blood–brain barrier (BBB) by way of endothelial damage.[6]

Because the tissue pathophysiology of acute ischemic stroke is closely linked with water content, MR imaging modalities are powerful diagnostic tools to identify and age ischemia and ultimately to provide valuable tissue level information. Diffusion weighted imaging (DWI) and apparent diffusion coefficient (ADC) are highly sensitive for detecting acute ischemia, and abnormalities can emerge as early as minutes from the onset of stroke symptoms.[7] With time, vasogenic edema begins to accumulate, and fluid attenuated inversion recovery (FLAIR) abnormalities begin to emerge.[8] Eventually, BBB breakdown occurs, leading to contrast extravasation on contrast-enhanced sequences.[9] The time course and appearance of DWI, ADC, FLAIR, and contrast signal abnormalities during early and late AIS are presented in Figs. 1 and 2.

It is important to note that although DWI and ADC abnormalities are sensitive markers of cytotoxic edema secondary to acute ischemia, they do not necessarily imply tissue death or infarction.[10] In fact, lesions harboring DWI and ADC abnormalities can normalize without subsequent evidence of irreversible tissue damage in other brain pathologic conditions such as seizures and cerebral venous thromboses.[11] DWI lesions in acute ischemic stroke are also thought to be somewhat reversible after restoration of blood flow.[12] Although some DWI/ADC lesions can be reversible, substantial signal changes are likely indicative of nonsalvageable ischemic tissue (also termed ischemic core),[13] and an ADC value of less than 620×10^{-6} mm^2/s is generally accepted as a threshold to identify irreversible damage.[14] Another possible marker for irreversible damage is the presence of FLAIR abnormalities. Given that vasogenic edema generally develops as a delayed process secondary to acute ischemia, FLAIR abnormalities normally emerge at least 3 hours following stroke onset (see Fig. 2).[5] Presence of FLAIR lesions is significantly associated with worse clinical outcomes following recanalization therapy.[15] Thus, studies have proposed the use of FLAIR abnormalities as a form of "tissue clock," where the absence of FLAIR lesions may indicate relatively acute ischemia, and presence of FLAIR lesions may indicate progression to tissue death.[16]

MR IMAGING TO CHARACTERIZE VESSELS AND HEMODYNAMICS

In addition to characterizing tissue status for patients with acute ischemic stroke, MR techniques can also accurately assess status of the cerebral vasculature and their hemodynamics to guide recanalization therapy. To assess the patency of intracranial vessels, time-of-flight (TOF) angiography can be used to localize the site of vascular occlusion. This technique capitalizes on the entry of unsaturated spins flowing into imaging slices with saturated and stational spins, and it does not require the administration of gadolinium contrast.[17] Although TOF angiography is sensitive in identifying large vessel occlusions, vessels with slow or turbulent flow may result in signal loss, which may lead to misclassification of partially patent vessels as occluded[18] (Fig. 3). Furthermore, the lengthy acquisition time of TOF angiography makes patient cooperation a limiting factor, and visualization of medium or smaller vessels can be challenging.[17] Thus, although uncommonly used, addition of gadolinium contrast-enhanced angiography may overcome some of these limitations.[19] In addition to identifying sites of vascular occlusion in acute ischemic stroke, MR angiography techniques can also be used to identify other vascular abnormalities (eg, atherosclerotic disease,[20] dissection,[21]

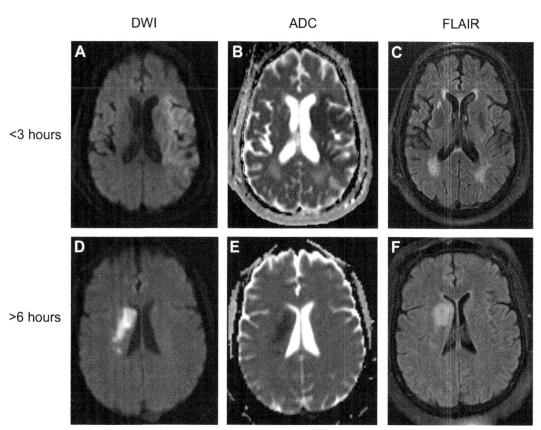

	DWI	ADC	FLAIR
<3 hours	A	B	C
>6 hours	D	E	F

Fig. 2. (A–F) MR imaging findings for acute ischemic in the hyperacute (<4.5 hours from onset) and early subacute (6 or more hours from onset). Specifically, FLAIR is generally silent during hyperacute stroke (C), and FLAIR hyperintense lesions start to seem as ischemia progresses to infarction (F).

and so forth) that may provide important information regarding stroke cause. The clots themselves can also be visualized on susceptibility-weighted or gradient echo sequences,[22] which can be useful when angiography does not clearly demonstrate occlusion of branch vessels that may occur at the origin (Fig. 4), and may also provide additional information that may be valuable for treatment planning.[23]

Identification and quantification of hypoperfused but not yet unsalvageable tissue (also termed the stroke penumbra) is a key tenant of acute stroke triage, and the penumbra is classically considered the treatment target of endovascular therapy, especially in extended time windows.[24] The most common method for identifying hypoperfusion is perfusion-weighted imaging (PWI) and their associated time metrics of gadolinium contrast transit in oligemic or ischemic tissue (eg, time to peak [TTP], mean transit time, and so forth).[25] In conjunction with ADC, abnormal PWI metrics can be used to identify the stroke penumbra, which is generally defined as TTP values greater than 6 seconds with ADC signals of

620×10^{-6} mm^2/s or higher (Fig. 5).[14,26] Arterial spin labeling (ASL) is another perfusion technique that labels water spins in the cervical vessels with an inversion impulse and then following a delay captures the desired volume.[27] ASL has an advantage of not requiring the use of gadolinium contrast; however, it only permits the quantification of cerebral blood flow, and it cannot measure other perfusion metrics (cerebral blood volume [CBV], TTP, and time-to-maximum [Tmax]), thereby limiting its use in acute ischemic stroke imaging.[27] Hypointensity of subependymal and deep medullary veins in susceptible-weighted or gradient-echo (GRE) sequences (brush sign) has also been associated with hypoperfused tissue.[28] Finally, FLAIR hyperintense vessels are also associated with stagnant flow, and their presence is associated with the volume of hypoperfused tissue as well (see Fig. 3C).[29,30]

MR perfusion studies can also provide useful clinical information after acute stroke treatment and recanalization for vascular occlusions. Past studies have shown that some of the tissue may not stay well perfused as evidenced by perfusion

CT Angiography

FLAIR

TOF MRA

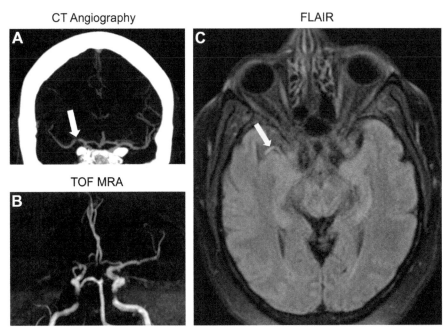

Fig. 3. (A–C) Although CTA (A) demonstrates vessel stenosis (*white arrow*) with distal reconstitution of flow, TOF angiography (B) may suggest vessel occlusion. Vessels with slow flow can present as hyperintense on FLAIR (C, *yellow arrow*).

studies, despite complete vascular recanalization (also termed "no-reflow" phenomenon), which was associated with worse clinical outcomes.[31] Hyperemia of reperfused tissue can also occur, which has also been associated with lesion growth and poor outcomes.[32] Thus, MR perfusion studies after acute ischemic stroke may yield helpful clinical information after stroke recanalization, and the use of perfusion metrics as biomarkers for new stroke therapies awaits future research.

GRE

TOF MRA

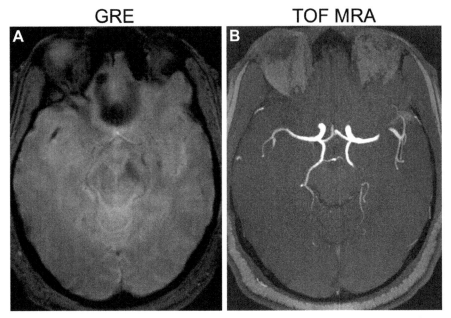

Fig. 4. (A, B) Demonstration of GRE positive clot in an M2 segment of the right middle cerebral artery without clear visualization of vascular occlusion in TOF MR angiogram (B).

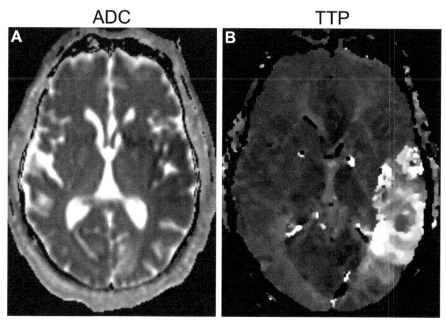

ADC   TTP

Fig. 5. (A, B) Demonstration of core (A) and perfusion (B) mismatch suggesting presence of stroke penumbra and possibly salvageable tissue.

MR IMAGING VERSUS COMPUTED TOMOGRAPHY FOR ACUTE STROKE TRIAGE

There are several advantages and disadvantages to both MR and computed tomography (CT) imaging for acute stroke triage. Although MR imaging allows for far superior tissue characterization than CT imaging, studies take longer than CT, and they are also costlier financially. Past studies have shown that MR-based ischemic stroke triage can achieve comparable time efficiency as CT[33]; however, CT remains the mainstay imaging modality worldwide due to its widespread availability and relatively lower cost. Thus, despite the advantages inherent to MR imaging for ischemic strokes, institutions that use MR-based acute stroke triage systems remain a minority worldwide.

One important advantage of MR-based acute stroke triage is the ability of MR to reliable identify early acute ischemia. The initial landmark IVT trials for acute ischemic stroke did not rely on identifying tissue ischemia, and to be eligible, patients would only need a clinical diagnosis of stroke with measurable neurologic deficit presenting within a stringent time window (less than 4.5 hours from time of last known normal).[34,35] CT imaging was used mainly to rule out intracranial hemorrhage, established infarct, or other intracranial abnormalities but it provided little additional value because most stroke patients who would benefit from treatment would have no abnormalities on CT. Because MR imaging can identify acute ischemia within

minutes of stroke onset, presence or absence of DWI lesions can be used to better evaluate patients with mild neurologic symptoms to rule out stroke mimics.[36] It can also be used to provide additional diagnostic confidence for posterior circulation strokes that may present with nonspecific neurologic symptoms such as dizziness, vertigo, diplopia, or other cranial nerve abnormalities.[37]

MR imaging can also be used during acute triage to assess DWI-FLAIR mismatch to expand eligibility for thrombolysis. Presence of DWI/ADC abnormalities in the absence of FLAIR lesions is indicative of relatively acute ischemia, and the MR WITNESS[38] and WAKE-UP[39] trials showed that IV thrombolysis for these patients is effective and safe. Thus, an MR-based acute stroke triage system may be helpful for expanding acute stroke treatment of patients presenting with unknown time of stroke onset or extended time from last-known-normal. DWI-clinical mismatch, as detailed in the DAWN trial,[40] can also be used to determine eligibility for extended time-window EVT. Using DWI-clinical mismatch obviates any intravenous contrast agent, which may be advantageous for patients with contrast allergies or difficult vascular access. Furthermore, diffusion sequences with MR do not rely on perfusion metrics; thus, MR is a more direct tool to assess tissue ischemia and may be more reliable in quantifying ischemic cores with patients with underlying stenotic disease or poor cardiac output than perfusion metrics. For patients with high clinical suspicion for large vessel occlusion (eg, patients with high VAN[41] or LAMS[42] scores), an abbreviated MR imaging protocol with a diffusion sequence, a susceptibility-weighted or gradient echo sequence, and MR angiography can be accomplished within 10 minutes to provide all necessary information for making treatment decisions for EVT.

Another advantage of using MR imaging for acute stroke triage is to aid in the treatment decision for minor strokes. Although the results of the PRISMS[43] and ARAMIS[44] trials suggest that thrombolysis may not be effective for minor stroke patients without disabling deficits compared with antiplatelet therapy alone, most of the trial participants went through CT-based triage systems, and as such, the study population may have been enriched with stroke mimics who would not benefit from thrombolysis. In this respect, whether patients with minor strokes that have measurable abnormalities on diffusion-weighted MR imaging would benefit from thrombolysis is unclear and future research is needed.[45]

Susceptibility-weighted or gradient echo sequences can also be used to identify cerebral microbleeds, which can be valuable information to optimize thrombolysis treatment decisions for patients with minor strokes.[46] One uncommon but devastating consequence of thrombolytic treatment of acute ischemic stroke is intraparenchymal hemorrhage outside the acutely ischemic tissue, and presence of microbleeds is a potential predictor. Studies have shown that cerebral microbleed burden is significantly associated with higher rates of symptomatic intracranial hemorrhage following thrombolysis. Thus, having 10 microbleeds or more on susceptibility-weighted or gradient echo sequences can be considered a relative contraindication to thrombolysis, especially in older patients and those experiencing treatment delays.[46]

Finally, with ever improving treatment modalities and patient eligibility, differentiation of salvageable and unsalvageable tissue at the time of acute stroke triage is increasingly important. Although both MR and CT techniques use similar methods to identify areas of hypoperfusion by using time metrics of contrast transit through ischemic or oligemic tissue, MR's excellent ability to identify and quantify ischemic cores with DWI and ADC abnormalities is likely superior to CT. Currently, there are 2 methods to quantify the ischemic core on CT: the ASPECT score[47] and CT perfusion imaging.[48,49] The ASPECT score is used to quantify areas of the brain that are exhibiting signs of early ischemia (eg, loss of gray white matter differentiation, sulcal effacement, hypodensity, and so forth), and it has served as an exclusion criterion for many of the landmark thrombectomy trials.[50] However, several recent studies demonstrated that thrombectomy is safe and may still yield benefit in patients with low ASPECT scores,[51,52] which may reflect ASPECT's low positive predictive value of true ischemic core. CT perfusion imaging, namely relative cerebral blood flow, has also been used to quantify ischemic core in clinical trials.[48,49] However, this method is also prone to inaccuracies. For example, CT perfusion may erroneously overestimate ischemic cores, a phenomenon termed "ghost infarct core."[53] The converse may also occur; in DEFUSE-3, a study of thrombectomy for late-window patients using perfusion imaging, patients who underwent MR-based selection fared better than patients who underwent CT-based selection, which could suggest that CT-based methods of estimating ischemic core may underestimate true infarct volume compared with MR-based protocols.[51] Future studies are needed to further investigate the importance of ischemic core quantification for acute stroke treatment decisions as well as the clinical value of MR's superiority in this regard.

MR IMAGING FOR THE IDENTIFICATION AND QUANTIFICATION OF HEMORRHAGIC TRANSFORMATION OF ACUTE ISCHEMIC STROKE

Hemorrhagic transformation of acute ischemic strokes is a common sequela, and prompt identification can guide the optimization of blood pressure control and use of poststroke anithrombotic medications.[54] The original classification system was described by European Cooperative Acute Stroke Study (ECASS-II),[55] which used CT imaging to identify hemorrhage; hemorrhagic transformations are categorized into scattered petechial hemorrhage (HI-1), confluent petechial hemorrhage (HI-2), parenchymal hematoma that occupies 30% or less of the ischemic bed (PH-1), and parenchymal hematoma that occupies more than 30% of the ischemic bed (PH-2). More recently, the Heidelberg classification system expanded on the initial European-Australasian Acute Stroke Study (ECASS) system by including intraventricular hemorrhage, SAH, subdural hematoma, and intraparenchymal hemorrhage outside acute ischemic tissue.[56]

Although GRE and susceptibility-weighted sequences can reliably identify hemorrhagic transformations, the nature of blooming artifacts can exaggerate the appearance of bleeds.[57] Importantly, most studies that established the impact hemorrhagic transformations have on clinical outcomes that shaped current practice were done with CTs.[58] Thus, providers should remember that MR imaging may be significantly more sensitive than CTs for identifying hemorrhages and that they should be interpreted with relative caution. In addition to GRE and susceptibility-weighted sequences, MR is also able to leverage the changes in paramagnetism of hemoglobin molecules over time to age blood, which may be helpful information for patients presenting with unknown time of stroke or hemorrhage onset.[59]

MR imaging can also be used to assess BBB integrity. The hyperacute injury marker (HARM) is characterized by sulcal or ventricular enhancement of postcontrast FLAIR sequences, and it may be a marker of BBB disruption.[60] Studies have demonstrated that presence of HARM may help in the prediction of hemorrhagic transformations and guide blood pressure management for stroke patients.[61] Future studies are needed to further validate its clinical utility before routine use.

MR IMAGING FOR THE DIAGNOSIS AND CHARACTERIZATION OF DELAYED CEREBRAL ISCHEMIA FOLLOWING SUBARACHNOID HEMORRHAGE

In addition to its central role in the diagnosis and management of acute ischemic stroke, MR imaging also has an important role in the identification and management of secondary ischemic injury due to SAH, commonly termed DCI.[62] Although the definition of DCI remains somewhat controversial, it is a generally accepted term to describe the phenomenon of ischemic damage to brain parenchyma occurring 72 or more hours after the onset of SAH, particularly aneurysmal SAH. The pathophysiological mechanism underlying DCI is complex and may involve multiple pathways including vasospasm,[63] endothelial damage and microthrombosis,[64] impaired cerebral autoregulation,[65] cortical spreading depolarization,[66] and inflammation and BBB disruption.[67]

Clinically, DCI normally manifests as new focal neurologic deficits with onset days after SAH; however, for critically ill patients with poor neurologic examinations, identification of DCI may be challenging and thus may rely on imaging techniques. Overall, MR provides important tissue-level information that other imaging modalities do not provide,[68,69] and despite lower spatial resolution, its multimodality and the excellent contrast resolution of DWI allows identification of new ischemic lesions regardless of their location and size (Fig. 6). In addition, MR imaging can also identify a variety of other pathologic conditions (eg, infection, hydrocephalus, and so forth) that may develop during the subacute phase of aSAH, particularly for patients who underwent surgical treatment.

MR ANGIOGRAPHY FOLLOWING SUBARACHNOID HEMORRHAGE

Cerebral vasospasm is a measurable, reversible, and prolonged narrowing of major cerebral arteries that can occur days after SAH,[64] and it is thought to play a central role in the pathophysiology of DCI. Transcranial Doppler ultrasound and CT angiography (CTA) are commonly used for screening and initial evaluation, and digital subtraction angiography (DSA) is the gold standard diagnostic tool. Although less commonly used, TOF angiography demonstrated acceptable sensitivity and specificity for identifying intracranial vasospasm.[70] Although detection of vasospasm using TOF angiography may be negatively impacted by the T1-hyperintensity of methemoglobin within early subacute blood from SAH, it may be less susceptible than CTA to artifacts in postsurgical or postembolization patients (Fig. 7). Other MR techniques, namely quantitative MRA,[71] have demonstrated the ability to quantify volume flow rate through cerebral vasculature in the setting of vasospasm, overall showing good correlation with DSA vessel diameters ($r_s = 0.71$, $P<.001$).[72] Vessel wall imaging (VWI) imaging can also provide useful information suggesting rupture site in patients with coexisting aneurysm and SAH. To date, 2 meta-analyses[73,74] have shown how vessel wall enhancement is associated with rupture while lack of it can predict aneurysm stability. Additional details regarding VWI will be discussed in a separate section of this issue.

MR PERFUSION FOLLOWING SUBARACHNOID HEMORRHAGE

Similar to their use for acute ischemic stroke, cerebral perfusion measurements can be performed with MR imaging during the subacute phase of SAH. Past studies have demonstrated that perfusion MR imaging findings can be used to guide treatment and predict outcomes.[75,76] Flow, volume, and time maps can be generated from gadolinium-based perfusion studies by measuring the loss of T2/T2* signals as contrast material perfuses cerebral tissue (dynamic susceptibility contrast, DSC). Hattingen and colleagues[77] showed how simultaneous decrease of relative cerebral blood flow (rCBF) and relative cerebral blood volume (rCBV), studied with DSC-MR imaging, can reflect the absence of relevant vasodilation and reveal early impairment in cerebral perfusion in vasospasm. Another, less commonly used, method to generate perfusion metrics is to measure increased T1 signals in the capillary bed dynamic contrast-enhanced (DCE). One key distinction and limit of DSC is that it assumes an intact BBB; therefore,

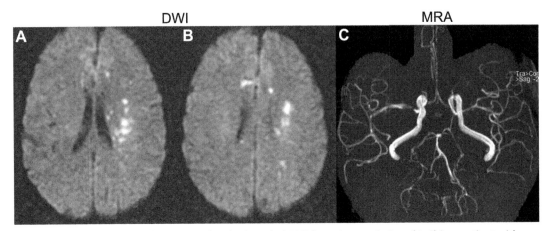

Fig. 6. (A–C) Demonstration of tiny cortical and subcortical DWI hyperintense lesions (A, B) in a patient with vasospasm (C).

MR perfusion metrics derived by DSC should be interpreted with caution. However, although DCE is computationally intensive, subtle BBB changes can be detected, and this information may be helpful in identifying patients at high risk for developing DCI.[78] ASL can also be used to identify perfusion deficits requiring urgent treatment[79]; however, because it is only able to capture flow metrics but not volume or time metrics, its use in patients with SAH is limited considering how often these patients have pharmacologically or physiologically altered cerebral autoregulation.

Intravascular incoherent motion (IVIM) is another less commonly used MR imaging perfusion technique that uses information derived from both DWI and ADC to calculate the fraction of water following perfused capillaries (f). Heit and colleagues[80] showed that decreased IVIM f is correlated with DCI and proximal arterial vasospasm. IVIM does not require contrast administration and has the advantage of only needing DWI and ADC to evaluate tissue perfusion.

In conclusion, quoting the ACR Appropriateness Criteria[81]: "Despite these positive studies, no large or prospective studies have been performed to support the widespread use of MR imaging perfusion in the evaluation of suspected vasospasm."

MR IMAGING FOR REVERSIBLE CEREBRAL VASOCONSTRICTION SYNDROME

In addition to its use for acute ischemic stroke and SAH, MR imaging is also a pillar in the diagnosis of other cerebral vasoconstricting entities such as reversible cerebral vasoconstriction syndrome (RCVS).

RCVS is a clinical syndrome characterized by recurrent episodes of sudden-onset headaches, with or without focal neurologic deficits; although not always present, neuroimaging often reveals diffuse, multifocal, and segmental arterial narrowing. Magnetic resonance angiography (MRA) can reveal RCVS's pathognomonic sign of segmental vasoconstriction, usually affecting large or medium

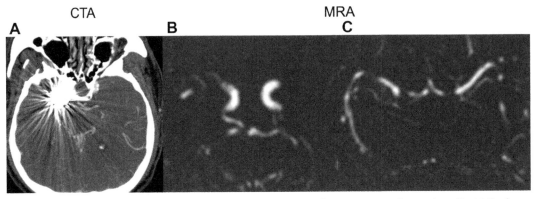

Fig. 7. (A–C) Findings in a patient with suspected vasospasm. CTA demonstrates coils streak artifact (A) whereas MRA exquisitely excludes it (B, C).

vessels. Vasoconstriction in RCVS is entirely reversible in most cases; however, neurologic injury due to SAH, intraparenchymal or subdural hemorrhage, and tissue ischemia may result in lasting clinical disability. Although DSC-MR imaging use has been reported,[82] it is not routinely used in clinical practice. Reduction of CBF measured by ASL has also been used for monitoring disease progression.[83] High spatial resolution sequences (VWI) can also be useful in the diagnosis demonstrating arterial wall thickening and enhancement[84] and will be discussed in a separate article (MR Vessel Wall Imaging for Atherosclerosis and Vasculitis) of the current issue.

SUMMARY

MR is a powerful tool for the diagnosis and quantification of ischemic brain lesions due to acute ischemic stroke or DCI following SAH. MR allows for excellent tissue characterization that can provide critical tissue-level insight that can be used to guide clinical care. As treatments for AIS and SAH continue to advance, development of novel MR-derived biomarkers may further facilitate the optimization of patient management.

CLINICS CARE POINTS

- Optimal patient selection and treatment decisions for acute recanalization and secondary stroke prevention rely on thorough evaluation of patient's clinical history, neurological exam, and multi-modality neuroimaging.

- Multimodality DWI, ADC and FLAIR imaging can be a valuable tool for tissue characterization in acute ischemic stroke.

- MR techniques can accurately assess the status of the cerebral vasculature and their hemodynamics to guide recanalization therapy, while MR perfusion can provide useful clinical information pre and post therapy.

- MR-based ischemic stroke triage can achieve comparable time efficiency as CT; however, CT remains the mainstay imaging modality worldwide due to its widespread availability and relatively lower cost.

- MR can easily identify and help manage Delayed Cerebral Ischemia (DCI) in the setting of subarachnoid hemorrhage (SAH).

- Identification of cerebral vasospasm with MR perfusion is still controversial and should be the aim of future studies.

DISCLOSURE

D. Gandhi reports grants from Microvention, the Focused Ultrasound Foundation, United States, the NIH, United States and University of Calgary, Canada/NoNo Therapeutics. All other authors declared no potential conflicts of interest with respect to the research, authorship, and/or publication of this article.

REFERENCES

1. Pu L, Wang L, Zhang R, et al. Projected Global Trends in Ischemic Stroke Incidence, Deaths and Disability-Adjusted Life Years From 2020 to 2030. Stroke 2023;54(5):1330–9.

2. Powers WJ, Rabinstein AA, Ackerson T, et al. Guidelines for the Early Management of Patients With Acute Ischemic Stroke: 2019 Update to the 2018 Guidelines for the Early Management of Acute Ischemic Stroke: A Guideline for Healthcare Professionals From the American Heart Association/American Stroke Association. Stroke 2019;50(12):e344–418.

3. Francoeur CL, Mayer SA. Management of delayed cerebral ischemia after subarachnoid hemorrhage. Crit Care 2016;20(1):277.

4. Beauchamp NJ, Barker PB, Wang PY, et al. Imaging of acute cerebral ischemia. Radiology 1999;212(2):307–24.

5. Dostovic Z, Dostovic E, Smajlovic D, et al. Brain Edema After Ischaemic Stroke. Med Arch 2016;70(5):339–41.

6. Candelario-Jalil E, Dijkhuizen RM, Magnus T. Neuroinflammation, Stroke, Blood-Brain Barrier Dysfunction, and Imaging Modalities. Stroke 2022;53(5):1473–86.

7. van Everdingen KJ, van der Grond J, Kappelle LJ, et al. Diffusion-weighted magnetic resonance imaging in acute stroke. Stroke 1998;29(9):1783–90.

8. Thomalla G, Rossbach P, Rosenkranz M, et al. Negative fluid-attenuated inversion recovery imaging identifies acute ischemic stroke at 3 hours or less. Ann Neurol 2009;65(6):724–32.

9. Karonen JO, Partanen PL, Vanninen RL, et al. Evolution of MR contrast enhancement patterns during the first week after acute ischemic stroke. AJNR Am J Neuroradiol 2001;22(1):103–11.

10. Kranz PG, Eastwood JD. Does diffusion-weighted imaging represent the ischemic core? An evidence-based systematic review. AJNR Am J Neuroradiol 2009;30(6):1206–12.

11. Mariajoseph FP, Sagar P, Muthusamy S, et al. Seizure-induced reversible MRI abnormalities in status epilepticus: A systematic review. Seizure 2021;92:166–73.

12. Yoo J, Choi JW, Lee SJ, et al. Ischemic Diffusion Lesion Reversal After Endovascular Treatment. Stroke 2019;50(6):1504–9.

13. Grant PE, He J, Halpern EF, et al. Frequency and clinical context of decreased apparent diffusion coefficient reversal in the human brain. Radiology 2001;221(1):43–50.

14. Purushotham A, Campbell BCV, Straka M, et al. Apparent diffusion coefficient threshold for delineation of ischemic core. Int J Stroke 2015;10(3): 348–53.

15. Kim Y, Luby M, Burkett NS, et al. Fluid-Attenuated Inversion Recovery Hyperintense Ischemic Stroke Predicts Less Favorable 90-Day Outcome after Intravenous Thrombolysis. Cerebrovasc Dis 2021; 50(6):738–45.

16. Aoki J, Sakamoto Y, Suzuki K, et al. Fluid-Attenuated Inversion Recovery May Serve As a Tissue Clock in Patients Treated With Endovascular Thrombectomy. Stroke 2021;52(7):2232–40.

17. Miyazaki M, Lee VS. Nonenhanced MR angiography. Radiology 2008;248(1):20–43.

18. Edelman RR, Koktzoglou I. Noncontrast MR angiography: An update. J Magn Reson Imaging 2019; 49(2):355–73.

19. Boujan T, Neuberger U, Pfaff J, et al. Value of Contrast-Enhanced MRA versus Time-of-Flight MRA in Acute Ischemic Stroke MRI. AJNR Am J Neuroradiol 2018;39(9):1710–6.

20. Liebeskind DS, Kosinski AS, Lynn MJ, et al. Noninvasive fractional flow on MRA predicts stroke risk of intracranial stenosis. J Neuroimaging 2015; 25(1):87–91.

21. Lévy C, Laissy JP, Raveau V, et al. Carotid and vertebral artery dissections: three-dimensional time-of-flight MR angiography and MR imaging versus conventional angiography. Radiology 1994;190(1): 97–103.

22. Park MG, Oh SJ, Baik SK, et al. Susceptibility-Weighted Imaging for Detection of Thrombus in Acute Cardioembolic Stroke. J Stroke 2016;18(1): 73–9.

23. Campbell BCV. Clot Length Assessment in Stroke Therapy Decisions. Stroke 2016;47(3):643–4.

24. Demeestere J, Wouters A, Christensen S, et al. Review of Perfusion Imaging in Acute Ischemic Stroke: From Time to Tissue. Stroke 2020;51(3):1017–24.

25. Copen WA, Schaefer PW, Wu O. MR perfusion imaging in acute ischemic stroke. Neuroimaging Clin N Am 2011;21(2):259–83, x.

26. Chalet L, Boutelier T, Christen T, et al. Clinical Imaging of the Penumbra in Ischemic Stroke: From the Concept to the Era of Mechanical Thrombectomy. Front Cardiovasc Med 2022;9:861913.

27. Chalela JA, Alsop DC, Gonzalez-Atavales JB, et al. Magnetic resonance perfusion imaging in acute ischemic stroke using continuous arterial spin labeling. Stroke 2000;31(3):680–7.

28. Payabvash S, Benson JC, Taleb S, et al. Prominent cortical and medullary veins on susceptibility-weighted images of acute ischaemic stroke. Br J Radiol 2016;89(1068):20160714.

29. Reyes D, Simpkins AN, Hitomi E, et al. Estimating Perfusion Deficits in Acute Stroke Patients Without Perfusion Imaging. Stroke 2022;53(11):3439–45.

30. Shang WJ, Chen HB, Shu LM, et al. The Association between FLAIR Vascular Hyperintensity and Stroke Outcome Varies with Time from Onset. AJNR Am J Neuroradiol 2019;40(8):1317–22.

31. Ter Schiphorst A, Charron S, Hassen WB, et al. Tissue no-reflow despite full recanalization following thrombectomy for anterior circulation stroke with proximal occlusion: A clinical study. J Cereb Blood Flow Metab 2021;41(2):253–66.

32. Luby M, Hsia AW, Lomahan CA, et al. Post-ischemic hyperemia following endovascular therapy for acute stroke is associated with lesion growth. J Cereb Blood Flow Metab 2023;43(6):856–68.

33. Shah S, Luby M, Poole K, et al. Screening with MRI for Accurate and Rapid Stroke Treatment: SMART. Neurology 2015;84(24):2438–44.

34. National Institute of Neurological Disorders and Stroke rt-PA Stroke Study Group. Tissue plasminogen activator for acute ischemic stroke. N Engl J Med 1995;333(24):1581–7.

35. Hacke W, Kaste M, Bluhmki E, et al. Thrombolysis with alteplase 3 to 4.5 hours after acute ischemic stroke. N Engl J Med 2008;359(13):1317–29.

36. Hand PJ, Kwan J, Lindley RI, et al. Distinguishing between stroke and mimic at the bedside: the brain attack study. Stroke 2006;37(3):769–75.

37. Merwick Á, Werring D. Posterior circulation ischaemic stroke. BMJ 2014;348:g3175.

38. Schwamm LH, Wu O, Song SS, et al. Intravenous thrombolysis in unwitnessed stroke onset: MR WITNESS trial results. Ann Neurol 2018;83(5):980–93.

39. Thomalla G, Simonsen CZ, Boutitie F, et al. MRI-Guided Thrombolysis for Stroke with Unknown Time of Onset. N Engl J Med 2018;379(7):611–22.

40. Nogueira RG, Jadhav AP, Haussen DC, et al. Thrombectomy 6 to 24 Hours after Stroke with a Mismatch between Deficit and Infarct. N Engl J Med 2018; 378(1):11–21.

41. Teleb MS, Ver Hage A, Carter J, et al. Stroke vision, aphasia, neglect (VAN) assessment-a novel emergent large vessel occlusion screening tool: pilot study and comparison with current clinical severity indices. J Neurointerv Surg 2017;9(2):122–6.

42. Noorian AR, Sanossian N, Shkirkova K, et al. Los Angeles Motor Scale to Identify Large Vessel Occlusion: Prehospital Validation and Comparison With Other Screens. Stroke 2018;49(3):565–72.

43. Khatri P, Kleindorfer DO, Devlin T, et al. Effect of Alteplase vs Aspirin on Functional Outcome for Patients With Acute Ischemic Stroke and Minor Nondisabling Neurologic Deficits: The PRISMS Randomized Clinical Trial. JAMA 2018;320(2):156–66.

44. Chen HS, Cui Y, Zhou ZH, et al. Dual Antiplatelet Therapy vs Alteplase for Patients With Minor Nondisabling Acute Ischemic Stroke: The ARAMIS Randomized Clinical Trial. JAMA 2023;329(24):2135–44.

45. Hsia AW, Luby ML, Leigh R, et al. Prevalence of Imaging Targets in Patients With Minor Stroke Selected for IV tPA Treatment Using MRI: The Treatment of Minor Stroke With MRI Evaluation Study (TIMES). Neurology 2021;96(9):e1301–11.

46. Schlemm L, Endres M, Werring DJ, et al. Benefit of Intravenous Thrombolysis in Acute Ischemic Stroke Patients With High Cerebral Microbleed Burden. Stroke 2020;51(1):232–9.

47. Gereda JE, Leung DY, Thatayatikom A, et al. Relation between house-dust endotoxin exposure, type 1 T-cell development, and allergen sensitisation in infants at high risk of asthma. Lancet 2000; 355(9216):1680–3.

48. Ma H, Campbell BCV, Parsons MW, et al. Thrombolysis Guided by Perfusion Imaging up to 9 Hours after Onset of Stroke. N Engl J Med 2019;380(19): 1795–803.

49. Albers GW, Marks MP, Kemp S, et al. Thrombectomy for Stroke at 6 to 16 Hours with Selection by Perfusion Imaging. N Engl J Med 2018;378(8):708–18.

50. Goyal M, Menon BK, van Zwam WH, et al. Endovascular thrombectomy after large-vessel ischaemic stroke: a meta-analysis of individual patient data from five randomised trials. Lancet 2016; 387(10029):1723–31.

51. Sarraj A, Hassan AE, Abraham MG, et al. Trial of Endovascular Thrombectomy for Large Ischemic Strokes. N Engl J Med 2023. https://doi.org/10. 1056/NEJMoa2214403.

52. Huo X, Ma G, Tong X, et al. Trial of Endovascular Therapy for Acute Ischemic Stroke with Large Infarct. N Engl J Med 2023. https://doi.org/10. 1056/NEJMoa2213379.

53. Boned S, Padroni M, Rubiera M, et al. Admission CT perfusion may overestimate initial infarct core: the ghost infarct core concept. J Neurointerv Surg 2017;9(1):66–9.

54. Hong JM, Kim DS, Kim M. Hemorrhagic Transformation After Ischemic Stroke: Mechanisms and Management. Front Neurol 2021;12:703258.

55. Larrue V, von Kummer RR, Müller A, et al. Risk factors for severe hemorrhagic transformation in ischemic stroke patients treated with recombinant tissue plasminogen activator: a secondary analysis of the European-Australasian Acute Stroke Study (ECASS II). Stroke 2001;32(2):438–41.

56. von Kummer R, Broderick JP, Campbell BCV, et al. The Heidelberg Bleeding Classification: Classification of Bleeding Events After Ischemic Stroke and Reperfusion Therapy. Stroke 2015;46(10):2981–6.

57. Arnould MC, Grandin CB, Peeters A, et al. Comparison of CT and three MR sequences for detecting and categorizing early (48 hours) hemorrhagic transformation in hyperacute ischemic stroke. AJNR Am J Neuroradiol 2004;25(6):939–44.

58. Yaghi S, Willey JZ, Cucchiara B, et al. Treatment and Outcome of Hemorrhagic Transformation After Intravenous Alteplase in Acute Ischemic Stroke: A Scientific Statement for Healthcare Professionals From the American Heart Association/American Stroke Association. Stroke 2017;48(12):e343–61.

59. Bradley WG. MR appearance of hemorrhage in the brain. Radiology 1993;189(1):15–26.

60. Kidwell CS, Burgess R, Menon R, et al. Hyperacute injury marker (HARM) in primary hemorrhage: a distinct form of CNS barrier disruption. Neurology 2011;77(19):1725–8.

61. Upadhyaya P, Mehta A, Luby M, et al. Good outcome associated with blood-brain barrier disruption and lower blood pressure after endovascular therapy. J Stroke Cerebrovasc Dis 2023;32(1): 106870.

62. Haisenleder DJ, Khoury S, Zmeili SM, et al. The frequency of gonadotropin-releasing hormone secretion regulates expression of alpha and luteinizing hormone beta-subunit messenger ribonucleic acids in male rats. Mol Endocrinol 1987;1(11):834–8.

63. Dankbaar JW, Rijsdijk M, van der Schaaf IC, et al. Relationship between vasospasm, cerebral perfusion, and delayed cerebral ischemia after aneurysmal subarachnoid hemorrhage. Neuroradiology 2009;51(12):813–9.

64. Vergouwen MDI, Vermeulen M, van Gijn J, et al. Definition of delayed cerebral ischemia after aneurysmal subarachnoid hemorrhage as an outcome event in clinical trials and observational studies: proposal of a multidisciplinary research group. Stroke 2010;41(10):2391–5.

65. Budohoski KP, Czosnyka M, Smielewski P, et al. Cerebral autoregulation after subarachnoid hemorrhage: comparison of three methods. J Cereb Blood Flow Metab 2013;33(3):449–56.

66. Lauritzen M, Dreier JP, Fabricius M, et al. Clinical relevance of cortical spreading depression in neurological disorders: migraine, malignant stroke, subarachnoid and intracranial hemorrhage, and traumatic brain injury. J Cereb Blood Flow Metab 2011;31(1):17–35.

67. Provencio JJ. Inflammation in subarachnoid hemorrhage and delayed deterioration associated with vasospasm: a review. Acta Neurochir Suppl 2013; 115:233–8.

68. Siironen J, Porras M, Varis J, et al. Early ischemic lesion on computed tomography: predictor of poor outcome among survivors of aneurysmal subarachnoid hemorrhage. J Neurosurg 2007;107(6): 1074–9.

69. Hokari M, Shimbo D, Uchida K, et al. Characteristics of MRI Findings after Subarachnoid Hemorrhage

and D-Dimer as a Predictive Value for Early Brain Injury. J Stroke Cerebrovasc Dis 2022;31(1):106073.

70. Grandin CB, Cosnard G, Hammer F, et al. Vasospasm after Subarachnoid Hemorrhage: Diagnosis with MR Angiography. AJNR Am J Neuroradiol 2000;21(9):1611–7.

71. Bae YJ, Jung C, Kim JH, et al. Quantitative Magnetic Resonance Angiography in Internal Carotid Artery Occlusion with Primary Collateral Pathway. J Stroke 2015;17(3):320–6.

72. Shah KA, White TG, Teron I, et al. Quantitative magnetic resonance angiography as an alternative imaging technique in the assessment of cerebral vasospasm after subarachnoid hemorrhage. Interv Neuroradiol 2022. https://doi.org/10.1177/15910199221138167. 15910199221138168.

73. Texakalidis P, Hilditch CA, Lehman V, et al. Vessel Wall Imaging of Intracranial Aneurysms: Systematic Review and Meta-analysis. World Neurosurg 2018; 117:453–8.e1.

74. Wang X, Zhu C, Leng Y, et al. Intracranial Aneurysm Wall Enhancement Associated with Aneurysm Rupture: A Systematic Review and Meta-analysis. Acad Radiol 2019;26(5):664–73.

75. Hertel F, Walter C, Bettag M, et al. Perfusion-weighted Magnetic Resonance Imaging in Patients with Vasospasm: A Useful New Tool in the Management of Patients with Subarachnoid Hemorrhage. Neurosurgery 2005;56(1):28.

76. Beck J, Raabe A, Lanfermann H, et al. Effects of balloon angioplasty on perfusion- and diffusion-weighted magnetic resonance imaging results and outcome in patients with cerebral vasospasm. J Neurosurg 2006;105(2):220–7.

77. Hattingen E, Blasel S, Dettmann E, et al. Perfusion-weighted MRI to evaluate cerebral autoregulation in aneurysmal subarachnoid haemorrhage. Neuroradiology 2008;50(11):929–38.

78. Russin JJ, Montagne A, D'Amore F, et al. Permeability imaging as a predictor of delayed cerebral ischemia after aneurysmal subarachnoid hemorrhage. J Cereb Blood Flow Metab 2018;38(6):973–9.

79. Labriffe M, Ter Minassian A, Pasco-Papon A, et al. Feasibility and validity of monitoring subarachnoid hemorrhage by a noninvasive MRI imaging perfusion technique: Pulsed Arterial Spin Labeling (PASL). J Neuroradiol 2015;42(6):358–67.

80. Heit JJ, Wintermark M, Martin BW, et al. Reduced Intravoxel Incoherent Motion Microvascular Perfusion Predicts Delayed Cerebral Ischemia and Vasospasm After Aneurysm Rupture. Stroke 2018;49(3):741–5.

81. Ledbetter LN, Burns J, Shih RY, et al. ACR Appropriateness Criteria® Cerebrovascular Diseases-Aneurysm, Vascular Malformation, and Subarachnoid Hemorrhage. J Am Coll Radiol 2021;18(11):S283–304.

82. Rosenbloom MH, Singhal AB. CT angiography and diffusion-perfusion MR imaging in a patient with ipsilateral reversible cerebral vasoconstriction after carotid endarterectomy. AJNR Am J Neuroradiol 2007;28(5):920–2.

83. Kano Y, Inui S, Uchida Y, et al. Quantitative arterial spin labeling magnetic resonance imaging analysis of reversible cerebral vasoconstriction syndrome: A case series. Headache 2021;61(4):687–93.

84. Chen CY, Chen SP, Fuh JL, et al. Vascular wall imaging in reversible cerebral vasoconstriction syndrome – a 3-T contrast-enhanced MRI study. J Headache Pain 2018;19(1):74.

MR Imaging-based Biomarker Development in Hemorrhagic Stroke Patients Including Brain Iron Quantification, Diffusion Tensor Imaging, and Phenomenon of Ultra-early Erythrolysis

Momodou G. Bah, MPH[a], Ehsan Dowlati, MD[b], Max Fleigner, BS[c],
Sravanthi Koduri, MD[b], Aditya Pandey, MD[b,d], Leanne Y. Lin, MD, MPHS[d],
Thomas L. Chenevert, PhD[d], Jonathan Troost, PhD[e], Guohua Xi, MD[b],
Richard Keep, PhD[b], Neeraj Chaudhary, MD[b,d,f,*]

KEYWORDS

- MR imaging biomarkers • ICH • SAH • Iron toxicity
- Hematomal and perihematomal iron concentration • White matter injury • Early erythrolysis
- Early and late brain injury

KEY POINTS

- This review article discusses the role of MR imaging-based biomarkers in understanding and managing hemorrhagic strokes, focusing on intracerebral hemorrhage (ICH) and aneurysmal subarachnoid hemorrhage.
- ICH is a severe type of stroke with high mortality and morbidity rates, primarily caused by the rupture of small blood vessels in the brain, resulting in hematoma formation.
- Secondary brain injury occurs due to perihematomal edema, inflammation, and the toxic effects of clot components.
- Despite ongoing research, prognosis for ICH remains suboptimal, with no proven treatments available.

[a] Michigan State University College of Human Medicine, Lansing, MI, USA; [b] Department of Neurosurgery, University of Michigan, Ann Arbor, MI 48109, USA; [c] Oakland University, William Beaumont School of Medicine, Detroit, MI, USA; [d] Department of Radiology, University of Michigan, Ann Arbor, MI 48109, USA; [e] Michigan Institute for Clinical and Health Research, University of Michigan, Ann Arbor, MI 48109, USA; [f] Department of Otorhinolaryngology, University of Michigan, Ann Arbor, MI 48109, USA
* Corresponding author. Department of Radiology, Michigan Medicine, 1500 E Medical Center Drive, Ann Arbor, MI 48109.
E-mail address: neerajc@med.umich.edu

Neuroimag Clin N Am 34 (2024) 215–224
https://doi.org/10.1016/j.nic.2024.01.001
1052-5149/24/© 2024 Elsevier Inc. All rights reserved.

INTRODUCTION

Intracerebral hemorrhage (ICH) is a severe type of stroke with high mortality and morbidity rates.[1] Annually, in the United States, ICH affects approximately 80,000 patients, leading to more than 30,000 deaths.[2-4] This condition typically originates from the rupture of small parenchymal arteries or arterioles, resulting in hematoma formation.[2] Primary brain injury in ICH is caused by mechanical disruption from accumulated blood, leading to increased intracranial pressure, and compression of local structures.[5] Notably, hematoma expansion, which can be suggested by a "spot sign" on computed tomography (CT) angiography, is a common occurrence.[5] Secondary brain injury after ICH also occurs with perihematomal edema, inflammation, and the toxic effects of clot components.[5-7] Despite ongoing research, both early and late prognoses for ICH remain suboptimal.[1,8]

Apart from decompressive craniotomy, the management of ICH is centered around supportive care in critical care settings and rehabilitation units. No treatment paradigm has been proven to statistically improve neurologic outcomes. In addition, other than hematoma size, there are no established noninvasive imaging markers that project the appropriate prognosis. This review describes the development of novel MR imaging-based objective markers that could help with an improved prognostic assessment in ICH.

Aneurysmal subarachnoid hemorrhage (aSAH) is another devastating condition with high mortality, especially in the first few days after aneurysm rupture.[9,10] The incidence of aSAH is approximately 9 per 100,000 person-years, and it results in ~30% mortality, with long-term cognitive deficits observed in 50% of survivors.[11-13] Compared with other types of stroke, aSAH predominantly affects a younger age group and imposes a significant economic burden due to the loss of productive employment.[14] The underlying pathologic mechanisms of SAH-induced brain injury are likely multifactorial, involving ischemia, direct neurotoxicity of blood-derived components such as hemoglobin, and inflammation due to both ischemia and blood-derived components.[15,16] Early diagnosis and treatment play pivotal roles in potentially reducing mortality after aSAH.[17]

ROLE OF IRON IN HEMORRHAGIC STROKE

ICH can lead to devastating consequences.[18] Survivors of the initial ictus often experience severe neurologic deficits due to secondary insults triggered by the hematoma within the brain parenchyma.[19] Although the hematoma gradually resolves in humans over several months, functional restoration is often incomplete.[19] Animal studies have shed light on the mechanisms leading to brain injury after ICH.[20] These mechanisms involve thrombin produced during clot formation and hemoglobin and its breakdown products released during erythrocyte lysis within the hematoma.[21-24] Iron, as a hemoglobin degradation product, plays a critical role in neurodegeneration in various disease states.[19,25,26] Excessive brain iron accumulation can lead to oxidative stress and the formation of free radicals.[27]

Perihematomal iron accumulation has been observed in early and subacute ICH-induced brain injury but it persists longer term. In animal ICH models, Perl's staining indicates iron-positive cells in the perihematomal zone as early as the first day after ICH but high levels of nonheme iron persist in the brain for at least a month.[19] Other studies have shown a nearly 14-fold increase in free iron levels in cerebrospinal fluid (CSF) on the third day after ICH and those remain elevated for at least 28 days in experimental models.[28] This increase in iron around the hematoma reflects erythrolysis within the hematoma and the release of hemoglobin and iron. The extent of erythrolysis has been shown to have bearing on the extent of iron accumulation in the surrounding brain tissue.[29]

The amount of iron in the tissue influences the degree of inflammation and cytokine-mediated toxicity. This increase in brain iron levels contributes to brain edema, oxidative stress, brain atrophy, and neurologic deficits following ICH.[4,22,26,30,31] Iron from the hematoma also affects white matter fiber integrity causing fluid accumulation and cytotoxicity. Despite the gradual resolution of the hematoma in humans, neurologic deficits in patients with ICH often prove to be permanent and disabling.[2] In animal models, iron chelators have shown promise in reducing ICH-induced brain edema, neuronal death, brain atrophy, and neurologic deficits.[26,31] However, further studies are required to determine the efficacy of iron chelators through randomized controlled trials.[32,33] To comprehensively interpret the effects of such interventions, a thorough comprehension of the natural history and clinical importance of iron overload is necessary. There is an unmet need for objective biomarkers to assess severity of the neuronal damage and predict extent of functional recovery with time. This can be fulfilled to some extent by being able to determine the proportional erythrolysis within hematoma and understand its influence on the concentration of iron in the surrounding tissue and the extent of white matter injury both within the hematoma and in the surrounding tissue.

TECHNIQUES FOR BRAIN IRON QUANTIFICATION

Neuroimaging plays a crucial role in advancing our understanding of ICH natural history, particularly concerning iron due to its paramagnetic properties. Despite growing evidence linking iron to neuronal damage following ICH, a reliable paradigm for accurately quantifying tissue iron load is lacking.

MR imaging has emerged as a promising tool for revealing hemorrhagic brain injuries due to its high sensitivity to iron-containing compounds. Tissues with higher iron content display hypointensity on spin-echo and gradient-echo T2-weighted images, owing to the paramagnetic effects of tissue-deposited iron causing signal inhomogeneity.[34] In various clinical conditions requiring repeated blood transfusions, such as thalassemia, iron deposition occurs in different tissues of the body, and MR imaging has been exploited to estimate visceral tissue iron levels.[35–37] However, a robust technique for quantifying iron in human brain using MR imaging is still being studied. Some noteworthy advances have been made in brain iron quantification using MR imaging-based techniques. Bilgic and colleagues demonstrated the feasibility of detecting iron levels in brain tissues through quantitative susceptibility mapping (QSM), specifically the field-dependent relaxation rate technique.[38] Preliminary clinical studies have also shown the ability to detect cerebral tissue iron in traumatic brain injury (TBI) cases using T2* magnetic field correlation on MR imaging.[39] Liu and colleagues demonstrated the detection of superparamagnetic iron oxide nanoparticles in brain tissue following blood–brain barrier disruption using R2* relaxivity maps.[40] Moreover, Sammet and colleagues developed a mathematical model to differentiate between ferritin and hemosiderin on MR imaging using agarose-phantom and multiple spin echo sequences.[41] Investigating a porcine ICH model with 7T MR imaging, Wu and colleagues correlated T2* sequences with hematoma size and histopathological evidence of tissue iron.[42] Their study confirmed ferric iron deposition within the brain parenchyma, demonstrating the potential of MR imaging, especially T2* or gradient echo sequences, in indicating tissue iron deposition in a clinical setting. Moreover, Wang and colleagues highlighted the reliability of QSM on T2* MR imaging scans for quantifying hematoma volume in patients with ICH using R2* relaxivity maps.[43] They concluded that this technique holds

promise in providing a robust calculation of hematoma volume.

Overall, neuroimaging techniques, particularly MR imaging-based methods, present promising avenues for noninvasive brain iron quantification, shedding light on the role of iron in various neurologic conditions, including ICH.

BRAIN IRON QUANTIFICATION IN INTRACEREBRAL HEMORRHAGE
Imaging Characteristics of a Hematoma on MR Imaging

The manifestation of hematomas on MR imaging is influenced by several factors, including the age of the hematoma, the status of hemoglobin (oxyhemoglobin and deoxyhemoglobin), and the integrity of red blood cells (RBCs).[44,45] Understanding these factors is crucial in interpreting the imaging findings accurately.

In an ICH, changes in T2* signal on MR imaging have been categorized into 4 phases: hyperacute, acute, late subacute, and chronic.[1] During the hyperacute stage, the signal shows iso/hyperintense signal on T2* sequences primarily due to the presence of oxyhemoglobin within the hematoma.[46] With the progression of time, the oxygenated hemoglobin turns into deoxyhemoglobin, which then becomes hypointense on T2* sequences. However, it is essential to note that T2*-weighted MR images of both animal model and human hematomas may seem inhomogeneous.[34] This heterogeneity originates due to the coexistence of intracellular and extracellular hemoglobin within the hematoma, plus a mixture of oxygenated and deoxygenated hemoglobin causing variations in T2* signal intensity.[1]

Perihematomal Iron Quantification Techniques on MR Imaging

MR imaging has emerged as a valuable tool for assessing perihematomal iron concentration in the context of ICH. The MR imaging-based quantification of iron provides important insights into the underlying pathologic processes following ICH. Hemoglobin, in its intracellular or extracellular form, plays a critical role in causing signal hypointensity on T2*-weighted sequences after ICH due to its susceptibility to induce signal inhomogeneity. Deoxygenated hemoglobin exerts a greater paramagnetic effect compared with its oxygenated counterpart, leading to the exposure of more iron molecules and subsequent signal distortion on MR sequences. Consequently, MR image analysis can be used to quantify perihematomal iron concentration effectively (Fig. 1A).[2,47]

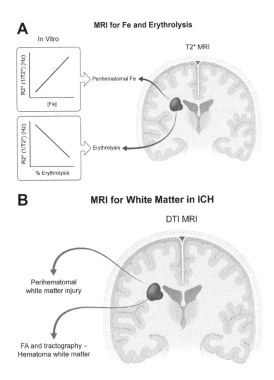

Fig. 1. The measurement of MR imaging parameters of iron and erythrolysis within and around the hematoma (*A*) and MR imaging parameters related to white matter tracts and its measurements are demonstrated in (*B*).

Several techniques have been used to measure perihematomal iron concentration. Researchers have used multiple echo train length and the Phase Difference Enhanced MR imaging sequence to measure the phase difference from iron in brain tissue.[1] Additionally, Relaxivity maps (R2*, which equals 1/T2*) have demonstrated promise in assessing perihematomal iron concentration because they reveal a near linear correlation with iron concentration.[1] To ensure accurate measurements, internal validation using measurements of iron-mediated signal phase difference on the hemisphere contralateral to ICH anatomic site is currently being explored by the authors in an NIH-funded study.[1]

Validation of MR imaging-based iron quantification has been conducted in both animal and human models. In a rat ICH model, the concept of measuring iron concentration through MR imaging signal magnitude calculations has been validated.[26] Encouragingly, human ICH measurements have also shown a good correlation with those obtained in porcine and rat ICH models.[47] Clinically, Wei and colleagues conducted a study to validate an MR imaging-based iron quantification algorithm in

humans.[8] Their approach involved assessing perihematomal iron concentration using R2* mapping on MR images and comparing the measurements to contralateral regions. The results revealed increased perihematomal iron concentrations after ICH, with peak elevation observed at days 3 and 14 followed by subsequent reduction to baseline levels by day 30.[8] Notably, the study also found a positive correlation between overall perihematomal iron overload and hematoma size, whereas no significant correlation was observed between perihematomal iron concentration and hematoma size (Fig. 2). In addition, perihematomal edema volume correlated with iron overload.[8] This study concluded that MR imaging with R2* mapping is an effective method to track tissue iron levels after ICH and highlights the correlations among iron overload, hematoma size, and edema volume.[8]

ULTRA-EARLY ERYTHROLYSIS IN INTRACEREBRAL HEMORRHAGE ON MR IMAGING
Definition and Characteristics of Ultra-early Erythrolysis

Hematoma lysis, hemoglobin release, and brain iron overload are significant contributors to brain injury after ICH.[4,48–51] The amount and rate of erythrolysis, defined as RBC breakdown and release of hemoglobin into the extracellular space, may be important factors determining iron exposure in perihematomal tissue.[23,52,53] For example, early erythrolysis, before iron defense mechanisms are upregulated, may be particularly harmful. However, the natural history of erythrolysis within the clot following ICH and the extent of early erythrolysis in the hematoma remain poorly examined.[44] Animal ICH models have demonstrated the proportion of "ghost" RBC (devoid of hemoglobin) correlating with proportional signal nonhypointensity on MR imaging. The same phenomenon has been depicted in human ICH. The rate of erythrolysis within the hematoma can have an impact on perihematomal iron levels after ICH.[44] Using MR imaging techniques such as T2* MR imaging and susceptibility-weighted imaging (SWI), the nonhypointensity of signal within the hematoma can be detected, which may serve as an indication of erythrolysis and extracellular degraded hemoglobin.[44]

Imaging Findings and MR Imaging Features of Early Erythrolysis

Early erythrolysis has been observed in both preclinical rat models and human patients with ICH, revealing intriguing MR imaging features. In a rat ICH model, areas with erythrocytes devoid of

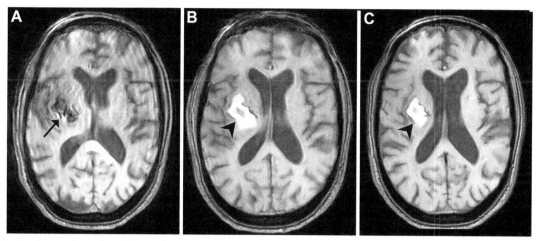

Fig. 2. Comparison of gradient echo sequence at 3 (*A*), 14 (*B*), and 30 (*C*) days after hemorrhage shows an initial drop in signal intensity and blooming artifact in regions of high iron concentration (*arrow*) but gradual increase in signal with erythrolysis (*arrowheads*).

intracellular hemoglobin were demonstrated by histology, which correlated with nonhypointense regions on T2* MR imaging within the hematoma.[44] Similarly, Wang and colleagues examined early erythrolysis in aged rats using MR imaging and found evidence of early erythrolysis within the hematoma after ICH.[54]

In patients with ICH, nonhypointense signals in the center of the hematoma were observed on T2*-weighted MR imaging at day 1, indicating the presence of early hemolysis.[34] The nonhypointense lesion volume increased significantly from day 1 to 14, and there was a linear correlation between the nonhypointense lesion volume and perihematomal edema volume at both time points, suggesting that early hemolysis significantly contributes to early brain edema in patients with ICH.[34]

Further investigations into the phenomenon of early erythrolysis were carried out by Novakovic and colleagues, who used MR imaging phantoms of pig blood with defined degrees of erythrolysis.[29] These phantoms demonstrated an excellent correlation between the percentage of erythrolysis and the R2* signal. The authors proposed that regions of T2* nonhypointensity within the hematoma can serve as a surrogate marker for early erythrolysis.

Gaining a comprehensive understanding of the imaging findings and MR imaging features of early erythrolysis holds significant importance in uncovering the influence of erythrolysis on ICH-induced brain injury. This knowledge may lead to the exploration of innovative therapeutic approaches with the aim of improving patient outcomes.

DIFFUSION TENSOR IMAGING IN INTRACEREBRAL HEMORRHAGE

Apart from adjacent gray matter, white matter fibers also exist in the region of the hematoma. Early brain injury from hematoma formation involves local destruction of gray and white matter tissue. White matter fibers may be sparsely preserved within the hematoma at the time of ictus. Animal model testing has shown that the existing integral white matter fibers following ICH acts as a scaffold for the migration of macrophages into the hematoma where they aid in hematoma resolution and the clearance of clot-derived factors such as hemoglobin and iron.[55]

MR imaging has the ability to track white matter fibers with preserved integrity in the human brain (Fig. 1B). Fractional anisotropy (FA) maps are generated from raw diffusion tensor imaging (DTI) data, which can be quantified. These are standard MR imaging sequences available on all MR imaging scanners currently used in clinical practice. The resolution of images obtained with DTI has increased and anatomic brain structures can be tracked more accurately.

Chen and colleagues demonstrated white matter fibers within the hematoma early after ICH (3 and 7 days) in the pig and these persisted up to 2 months following ictus.[55] In order to translate their animal model findings into human ICH analysis, the authors demonstrated similar phenomenon of relatively intact white matter fibers within the hematoma early on within 7 to 14 days after ICH (Fig. 3). The proportion of healthy white matter by FA quantification has been shown to increase with time to relatively normal levels in comparison

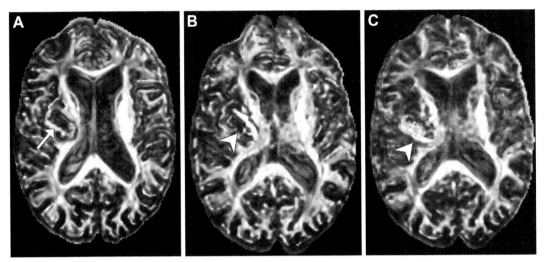

Fig. 3. Comparison of FA derived from DTI sequence at 3 (*A*), 14 (*B*), and 30 (*C*) days after hemorrhage shows initial drop in signal intensity in the hemorrhage (*arrow*) but gradual increase in signal over time (*arrowheads*).

to the contralateral white matter in an anatomically identical location in contralateral brain, by 30 days following ICH.[56]

BRAIN IRON QUANTIFICATION IN ANEURYSMAL SUBARACHNOID HEMORRHAGE
Quantitative Assessment of Iron in Patients with Aneurysmal Subarachnoid Hemorrhage

Imaging in the acute phase of aSAH may provide crucial insights into early brain injury caused by SAH.[57] Galea and colleagues conducted an imaging study to investigate whether iron deposition observed histologically in the gray matter persists beyond 2 weeks after aSAH and whether it correlates with clinical outcomes.[58] In 21 patients with aSAH, blood clot volume on admission CT was measured, and QSM using MR imaging was performed at 6 months after ictus. The study confirmed the presence of gray matter iron deposition at 6 months after aSAH, with the magnitude and laterality of iron deposition correlated to the blood clot volume on admission CT. Magnetic susceptibility, as measured by SWI, demonstrated a strong correlation with iron content.[58]

The use of quantitative imaging techniques to assess brain iron deposition in patients with aSAH provides valuable insights into the potential long-term effects of the initial hemorrhage on cognitive outcomes. Furthermore, the presence of heme metabolites such as ferritin has been shown to be significantly increased in aSAH with chronic hydrocephalus needing permanent CSF diversion.[59] This is also correlated with worse functional outcomes in these patients at 3 months.[59] Although such

observations may not denote causation, the ability to reduce ferritin burden after aSAH may reduce shunt dependency. By understanding the relationship between iron deposition and clinical outcomes, we may uncover new avenues for targeted interventions to improve the prognosis and quality of life for individuals affected by aSAH.

With iron quantification becoming a promising imaging marker for functional outcome, it provides a potential point of intervention by reducing iron burden for these patients. Deferoxamine has been shown to reduce mortality in a rat SAH model.[60] The authors are currently undertaking a randomized controlled trial evaluating the effects of deferoxamine in aSAH on imaging and functional outcomes.

Use of Diffusion Tensor Imaging in Patients with Aneurysmal Subarachnoid Hemorrhage

The use of DTI to evaluate white matter tracts in aSAH has been shown to be of prognostic use in predicting motor function and mortality in animal and human models, respectively.[61] Changes in DTI parameters are not yet well defined in aSAH imaging but do show promise as an imaging marker for outcome or point of intervention. These changes seem to be dynamic because there are changes in FA and augmented diffusion co-efficient (ADC) over time from the acute period to weeks after ictus.[62] In the acute setting, decreased FA values within 72 hours of ictus have been shown to be an independent marker of delayed cerebral ischemia in patients with aSAH.[63] In the subacute setting (within 8–10 days after ictus), Fragata and colleagues demonstrated that increased ADC values at the frontal centrum semiovale and decreased

FA at the corpus callosum are independently associated with worse functional outcomes.[64] The use of DTI is better established in severe TBI where studies have demonstrated white matter loss after TBI, suggesting structural disconnections, are associated with poor outcome and long-term disability.[65] Similarly, a study evaluating DTI parameters in both patients with severe TBI and high-grade aSAH demonstrated that lower FA values correlated with mortality.[66] In other clinical studies, patients with aSAH have been shown to have lower FA values within the corticospinal tracts of the midbrain compared with healthy controls 4 weeks after ictus[67] as well as higher mean diffusivity in the acute setting.[68] However, neither of these studies demonstrated a correlation with motor function scores pointing to the fact that there are mechanisms at play that determine function other than white matter tracts. Scherfler and colleagues demonstrated that iron deposition within white matter and lower FA in tracts adjacent to the cingulate gyrus correlated with lower executive function in 14 SAH patients at 1 year after ictus compared with healthy controls. Interestingly, these imaging differences were not detected at 3 weeks after ictus.[69] Further studies are needed to delineate clinically significant changes in DTI parameters in the aSAH population and how this will affect outcomes. However, as availability and resolution improve for MR-based DTI imaging, this tool may provide valuable information in the acute and long-term setting for patients with aSAH as well as guide prognosis and management for these patients because it relates to mortality, delayed cerebral ischemia, or executive and/or motor functional recovery.

CLINICAL APPLICATIONS AND FUTURE PERSPECTIVES

Brain iron quantification, ultra-early erythrolysis, and DTI have emerged as potential biomarkers for hemorrhagic stroke, offering promising applications in various aspects of clinical management. These biomarkers hold the potential to facilitate early diagnosis, risk stratification, monitoring treatment response, and tracking disease progression. By using reliable MR-based iron quantification algorithms, clinicians can gain valuable insights into the severity of neurotoxicity and efficacy of iron-chelating agents such as deferoxamine in patients with ICH. Additionally, the correlation of brain tissue iron levels with functional outcomes may allow for predicting prognosis of ICH in patients in the future.[2]

T2*-weighted MR imaging scans have shown promise in detecting heme deposition and secondary damage after stroke, and they hold potential as a noninvasive method to study the evolution of iron deposition in the brain parenchyma surrounding ICH. This imaging technique can provide valuable information on interventions aimed at reducing iron deposition, and the extent of T2* changes can serve as a marker of chronic brain injury.[42]

MR imaging-based evaluations offer enhanced granularity in assessing hematoma size and surrounding edema. Novakovic and colleagues highlighted the robustness of MR imaging-based assessment in analyzing various markers of tissue toxicity, including perihematomal iron overload and white matter loss.[56] Furthermore, MR imaging can be correlated with cellular events such as erythrolysis occurring within the hematoma and the hematoma size, providing a comprehensive understanding of the pathophysiology and clinical implications of hemorrhagic stroke.[70] Novakovic and colleagues have also demonstrated the methodology of white matter analysis providing a noninvasive assessment of white matter integrity within and around the hematoma.[56] Increased proportion of healthy white matter during ICH healing could hypothetically correlate with improved functional outcome. Having means to objectively and noninvasively assess the temporal evolution after ICH could prove to be significantly influential in the management of these patients with ICH. The integration of brain iron quantification, proportional ultra-early erythrolysis, and healthy white matter as objective noninvasive biomarkers has the potential to greatly enhance the management and prognosis of hemorrhagic stroke patients, fostering better informed clinical decision-making and eventually improving patient outcomes.

SUMMARY

The application of MR imaging-multiparametric biomarker development based on iron quantification techniques, ultra-early erythrolysis, and white matter tract health assessment as objective markers in ICH studies holds significant promise. Detecting increased tissue iron levels using MR imaging provides a potential means to objectively monitor the effectiveness of iron-chelating therapy and predict functional outcomes in patients with ICH in the future. Tracking hematoma volume, erythrolysis proportion, iron overload on surrounding brain tissue over time, including white matter integrity, may offer insights into the severity of the toxic impact on brain tissue and surviving white matter tracts. A larger analysis of these parameters in human ICH cohorts could establish robust surrogate markers of tissue injury. The insights gained from the above translational findings offer valuable natural history information on hemorrhagic stroke pathophysiology and present potential applications to inform clinical management in the future.

CLINICS CARE POINTS

- Randomized clinical trials have not shown benefit of hematoma evacuation in ICH.
- MRI biomarkers may give insight into better selection of patients for evacuation.
- MRI could improve risk stratification in ICH.

FUNDING

This study was in part supported by grants from the National Institutes of Health: NS116786, NS10674, NS108042, NS099684, NS104663-02, and NS131514-01A1.

ETHICS APPROVAL FOR CASE REPORT

Institution Review Board (IRB) approval was waived because the university does not require IRB approval for this review.

ACKNOWLEDGMENTS

I would like to acknowledge Dr Jonathan Troost, PhD[e] for making substantial conceptual or design contributions.

DECLARATION OF CONFLICTING INTERESTS

The author(s) declared no potential conflicts of interest with respect to the research, authorship, and/or publication of this article.

REFERENCES

1. Chaudhary N, Pandey AS, Griauzde J, et al. Brain tissue iron quantification by MRI in intracerebral hemorrhage: Current translational evidence and pitfalls. J Cereb Blood Flow Metab 2019;39(3):562–4.
2. Chaudhary N, Pandey AS, Merchak K, et al. Perihematomal cerebral tissue iron quantification on MRI following intracerebral hemorrhage in two human subjects: proof of principle. Brain edema XVI: translate basic science into clinical practice 2016; 179–83.
3. Qureshi AI, Tuhrim S, Broderick JP, et al. Spontaneous intracerebral hemorrhage. N Engl J Med 2001;344(19):1450–60.
4. Xi G, Keep RF, Hoff JT. Mechanisms of brain injury after intracerebral haemorrhage. Lancet Neurol 2006;5(1):53–63.
5. Wilkinson DA, Pandey AS, Thompson BG, et al. Injury mechanisms in acute intracerebral hemorrhage. Neuropharmacology 2018;134(Pt B):240–8.
6. Hemphill JC 3rd, Bonovich DC, Besmertis L, et al. The ICH score: a simple, reliable grading scale for intracerebral hemorrhage. Stroke 2001;32(4):891–7.
7. Broderick JP, Grotta JC, Naidech AM, et al. The Story of Intracerebral Hemorrhage: From Recalcitrant to Treatable Disease. Stroke 2021;52(5):1905–14.
8. Wei J, Novakovic N, Chenevert TL, et al. Perihematomal brain tissue iron concentration measurement by MRI in patients with intracerebral hemorrhage. CNS Neurosci Ther 2020;26(9):896–901.
9. Etminan N. Aneurysmal subarachnoid hemorrhage-status quo and perspective. Transl Stroke Res 2015;6(3):167–70.
10. Macdonald RL, Pluta RM, Zhang JH. Cerebral vasospasm after subarachnoid hemorrhage: the emerging revolution. Nat Clin Pract Neurol 2007;3(5):256–63.
11. Broderick JP, Brott TG, Duldner JE, et al. Initial and recurrent bleeding are the major causes of death following subarachnoid hemorrhage. Stroke 1994;25(7):1342–7.
12. Mayer SA, Kreiter KT, Copeland D, et al. Global and domain-specific cognitive impairment and outcome after subarachnoid hemorrhage. Neurology 2002;59(11):1750–8.
13. de Rooij NK, Linn FH, van der Plas JA, et al. Incidence of subarachnoid haemorrhage: a systematic review with emphasis on region, age, gender and time trends. J Neurol Neurosurg Psychiatry 2007;78(12):1365–72.
14. Taylor TN, Davis PH, Torner JC, et al. Lifetime cost of stroke in the United States. Stroke 1996;27(9):1459–66.
15. Al-Khindi T, Macdonald RL, Schweizer TA. Cognitive and functional outcome after aneurysmal subarachnoid hemorrhage. Stroke 2010;41(8):e519–36.
16. Bulters D, Gaastra B, Zolnourian A, et al. Haemoglobin scavenging in intracranial bleeding: biology and clinical implications. Nat Rev Neurol 2018;14(7):416–32.
17. Wang Z, Chen J, Toyota Y, et al. Ultra-early cerebral thrombosis formation after experimental subarachnoid hemorrhage detected on t2* magnetic resonance imaging. Stroke 2021;52(3):1033–42.
18. Wang J. Preclinical and clinical research on inflammation after intracerebral hemorrhage. Prog Neurobiol 2010;92(4):463–77.
19. Wu J, Hua Y, Keep RF, et al. Iron and iron-handling proteins in the brain after intracerebral hemorrhage. Stroke 2003;34(12):2964–9.
20. Xi G, Keep RF, Hoff JT. Pathophysiology of brain edema formation. Neurosurgery Clinics 2002;13(3):371–83.

21. Lee KR, Colon GP, Betz AL, et al. Edema from intracerebral hemorrhage: the role of thrombin. J Neurosurg 1996;84(1):91–6.

22. Xi G, Wagner KR, Keep RF, et al. Role of blood clot formation on early edema development after experimental intracerebral hemorrhage. Stroke 1998; 29(12):2580–6.

23. Xi G, Keep RF, Hoff JT. Erythrocytes and delayed brain edema formation following intracerebral hemorrhage in rats. J Neurosurg 1998;89(6):991–6.

24. Huang F-P, Xi G, Keep RF, et al. Brain edema after experimental intracerebral hemorrhage: role of hemoglobin degradation products. J Neurosurg 2002;96(2):287–93.

25. Thompson KJ, Shoham S, Connor JR. Iron and neurodegenerative disorders. Brain Res Bull 2001; 55(2):155–64.

26. Hua Y, Nakamura T, Keep RF, et al. Long-term effects of experimental intracerebral hemorrhage: the role of iron. J Neurosurg 2006;104(2):305–12.

27. Siesjö B, Agardh C-D, Bengtsson F. Free radicals and brain damage. Cerebrovascular and brain metabolism reviews 1989;1(3):165–211.

28. Wan S, Hua Y, Keep RF, et al. Deferoxamine reduces CSF free iron levels following intracerebral hemorrhage. Acta Neurochir Suppl 2006;96:199–202.

29. Novakovic N, Wilseck ZM, Chenevert TL, et al. Assessing early erythrolysis and the relationship to perihematomal iron overload and white matter survival in human intracerebral hemorrhage. CNS Neurosci Ther 2021;27(10):1118–26.

30. Lee KR, Kawai N, Kim S, et al. Mechanisms of edema formation after intracerebral hemorrhage: effects of thrombin on cerebral blood flow, blood-brain barrier permeability, and cell survival in a rat model. J Neurosurg 1997;86(2):272–8.

31. Nakamura T, Keep RF, Hua Y, et al. Deferoxamine-induced attenuation of brain edema and neurological deficits in a rat model of intracerebral hemorrhage. J Neurosurg 2004;100(4):672–8.

32. Selim M, Yeatts S, Goldstein JN, et al. Safety and tolerability of deferoxamine mesylate in patients with acute intracerebral hemorrhage. Stroke 2011; 42(11):3067–74.

33. Selim M, Foster LD, Moy CS, et al. Deferoxamine mesylate in patients with intracerebral haemorrhage (i-DEF): a multicentre, randomised, placebo-controlled, double-blind phase 2 trial. Lancet Neurol 2019;18(5):428–38.

34. Liu R, Li H, Hua Y, et al. Early hemolysis within human intracerebral hematomas: an MRI study. Transl Stroke Res 2019;10(1):52–6.

35. Brittenham GM, Badman DG, National Institute of Diabetes and Digestive and Kidney Diseases NIDDKWorkshop. Noninvasive measurement of iron: report of an NIDDK workshop. Blood 2003; 101(1):15–9.

36. He T, Gatehouse PD, Anderson LJ, et al. Development of a novel optimized breathhold technique for myocardial T2 measurement in thalassemia. J Magn Reson Imag 2006;24(3):580–5.

37. Jensen PD. Evaluation of iron overload. Br J Haematol 2004;124(6):697–711.

38. Bilgic B, Pfefferbaum A, Rohlfing T, et al. MRI estimates of brain iron concentration in normal aging using quantitative susceptibility mapping. Neuroimage 2012;59(3):2625–35.

39. Raz E, Jensen JH, Ge Y, et al. Brain iron quantification in mild traumatic brain injury: a magnetic field correlation study. AJNR Am J Neuroradiol 2011; 32(10):1851–6.

40. Liu HL, Chen PY, Yang HW, et al. In vivo MR quantification of superparamagnetic iron oxide nanoparticle leakage during low-frequency-ultrasound-induced blood-brain barrier opening in swine. J Magn Reson Imag 2011;34(6):1313–24.

41. Sammet CL, Swaminathan SV, Tang H, et al. Measurement and correction of stimulated echo contamination in T2-based iron quantification. Magn Reson Imaging 2013;31(5):664–8.

42. Wu G, Xi G, Hua Y, et al. T2* magnetic resonance imaging sequences reflect brain tissue iron deposition following intracerebral hemorrhage. Transl Stroke Res 2010;1(1):31–4.

43. Wang S, Lou M, Liu T, et al. Hematoma volume measurement in gradient echo MRI using quantitative susceptibility mapping. Stroke 2013;44(8):2315–7.

44. Dang G, Yang Y, Wu G, et al. Early erythrolysis in the hematoma after experimental intracerebral hemorrhage. Transl Stroke Res 2017;8(2):174–82.

45. Bradley WG Jr. MR appearance of hemorrhage in the brain. Radiology 1993;189(1):15–26.

46. Macellari F, Paciaroni M, Agnelli G, et al. Neuroimaging in intracerebral hemorrhage. Stroke 2014;45(3): 903–8.

47. Haque ME, Gabr RE, Zhao X, et al. Serial quantitative neuroimaging of iron in the intracerebral hemorrhage pig model. J Cerebr Blood Flow Metabol 2018;38(3):375–81.

48. Keep RF, Hua Y, Xi G. Intracerebral haemorrhage: mechanisms of injury and therapeutic targets. Lancet Neurol 2012;11(8):720–31.

49. Xiong XY, Wang J, Qian ZM, et al. Iron and intracerebral hemorrhage: from mechanism to translation. Transl Stroke Res 2014;5(4):429–41.

50. Selim M, Sheth KN. Perihematoma edema: a potential translational target in intracerebral hemorrhage? Transl Stroke Res 2015;6(2):104–6.

51. Xiong XY, Yang QW. Rethinking the roles of inflammation in the intracerebral hemorrhage. Transl Stroke Res 2015;6(5):339–41.

52. Hua Y, Schallert T, Keep RF, et al. Behavioral tests after intracerebral hemorrhage in the rat. Stroke 2002;33(10):2478–84.

53. Song S, Hua Y, Keep RF, et al. A new hippocampal model for examining intracerebral hemorrhage-related neuronal death: effects of deferoxamine on hemoglobin-induced neuronal death. Stroke 2007; 38(10):2861–3.

54. Wang M, Hua Y, Keep RF, et al. Complement inhibition attenuates early erythrolysis in the hematoma and brain injury in aged rats. Stroke 2019;50(7):1859–68.

55. Chen J, Koduri S, Dai S, et al. Intra-hematomal white matter tracts act as a scaffold for macrophage infiltration after intracerebral hemorrhage. Transl Stroke Res 2021;12(5):858–65.

56. Novakovic N, Linzey JR, Chenevert TL, et al. White matter survival within and around the hematoma: quantification by MRI in patients with intracerebral hemorrhage. Biomolecules 2021;11(6). https://doi.org/10.3390/biom11060910.

57. Guo D, Wilkinson DA, Thompson BG, et al. MRI characterization in the acute phase of experimental subarachnoid hemorrhage. Transl Stroke Res 2017; 8(3):234–43.

58. Galea I, Durnford A, Glazier J, et al. Iron Deposition in the brain after aneurysmal subarachnoid hemorrhage. Stroke 2022;53(5):1633–42.

59. Suzuki H, Muramatsu M, Tanaka K, et al. Cerebrospinal fluid ferritin in chronic hydrocephalus after aneurysmal subarachnoid hemorrhage. J Neurol 2006;253(9):1170–6.

60. Lee JY, Keep RF, Hua Y, et al. Deferoxamine reduces early brain injury following subarachnoid hemorrhage. Acta Neurochir Suppl 2011;112:101–6.

61. Chaudhary N, Pandey AS, Gemmete JJ, et al. Diffusion tensor imaging in hemorrhagic stroke. Exp Neurol 2015;272:88–96.

62. Fragata I, Canhão P, Alves M, et al. Evolution of diffusion tensor imaging parameters after acute subarachnoid haemorrhage: a prospective cohort study. Neuroradiology 2017;59(1):13–21.

63. Fragata I, Alves M, Papoila AL, et al. Early prediction of delayed ischemia and functional outcome in acute subarachnoid hemorrhage: role of diffusion tensor imaging. Stroke 2017;48(8):2091–7.

64. Fragata I, Alves M, Papoila AL, et al. Prediction of clinical outcome in subacute subarachnoid hemorrhage using diffusion tensor imaging. J Neurosurg 2018;1–9.

65. Hellyer PJ, Leech R, Ham TE, et al. Individual prediction of white matter injury following traumatic brain injury. Ann Neurol 2013;73(4):489–99.

66. Sener S, Van Hecke W, Feyen BF, et al. Diffusion tensor imaging: a possible biomarker in severe traumatic brain injury and aneurysmal subarachnoid hemorrhage? Neurosurgery 2016;79(6):786–93.

67. Yeo SS, Choi BY, Chang CH, et al. Evidence of corticospinal tract injury at midbrain in patients with subarachnoid hemorrhage. Stroke 2012;43(8):2239–41.

68. Jang SH, Kwon YH. Midbrain injury in patients with subarachnoid hemorrhage: a diffusion tensor imaging study. Sci Rep 2022;12(1):187.

69. Scherfler C, Schiefecker AJ, Delazer M, et al. Longitudinal profile of iron accumulation in good-grade subarachnoid hemorrhage. Ann Clin Transl Neurol 2016;3(10):781–90.

70. Butcher KS, Baird T, MacGregor L, et al. Perihematomal edema in primary intracerebral hemorrhage is plasma derived. Stroke 2004;35(8):1879–85.

MR Imaging of the Cerebral Aneurysmal Wall for Assessment of Rupture Risk

Sebastian Sanchez, MD[a,1], Andres Gudino-Vega, MD[b], Katherine Guijarro-Falcon, MD[b], Jacob M. Miller, BSE[b], Luis E. Noboa, BA[c,1], Edgar A. Samaniego, MD, MS[b,d,e,*]

KEYWORDS

- Aneurysm vessel wall • Rupture risk • Aneurysm wall enhancement
- High-resolution vessel wall imaging

KEY POINTS

- High-resolution MR (HR-MR) imaging has been used to assess different characteristics of the aneurysm wall, such as thickness and enhancement after the administration of contrast gadolinium.
- Aneurysm wall enhancement has the potential to identify aneurysms at the risk of rupturing. Newer postacquisition processing tools such as 3-dimensional color mapping can quantify and characterize in detail the distribution of gadolinium enhancement within the aneurysm wall.
- HR-MR imaging has the potential to identify unstable aneurysms that may require treatment due to the high risk of rupture.
- HR-MR imaging coupled with other imaging techniques can be used to study aneurysms and assess the risk of rupture. These techniques include finite element analysis of the aneurysm wall, quantitative susceptibility mapping for the detection of micro-hemorrhage, and computational fluid dynamics. This multi-modality assessment aims at acquiring a better understanding of aneurysm biology to predict the risk of rupture.
- Radiomics and machine learning are among the new tools for analysis of brain aneurysms.

CURRENT ASSESSMENT OF THE RISK OF RUPTURE

The assessment of unruptured intracranial aneurysms (UIAs) poses significant challenges due to the limited understanding of their biology. Aneurysm size has long been regarded as a crucial factor in assessing the risk of rupture, with larger size often being correlated with a higher risk of rupture. The International Study of Unruptured Intracranial Aneurysms (ISUIA), involving 4060 patients, found that aneurysms larger than 7 mm were indeed associated with an increased risk of rupture.[1] However, a comprehensive meta-analysis of 12,609 aneurysms reported that most ruptured intracranial aneurysms (RIAs) were smaller than 7 mm in size.[2] Furthermore, a recent meta-analysis performed by the authors' group and involving 13,025 aneurysms reported an average size of 6.1 mm for RIAs. Interestingly, this analysis showed that the size of UIAs and RIAs may be similar in locations such as the anterior communicating artery.[3]

Recognizing the limitations of aneurysm size as the sole determinant of risk, researchers have explored alternative morphologic metrics for assessing the risk of rupture. Two of such metrics

[a] Department of Neurology, Yale University, LLCI 912, New Haven, CT 06520, USA; [b] Department of Neurology, University of Iowa, 200 Hawkins Drive, Iowa City, IA 52242, USA; [c] Universidad San Francisco de Quito, Quito, Ecuador; [d] Department of Neurosurgery, University of Iowa, 200 Hawkins Drive, Iowa City, IA 52242, USA; [e] Department of Radiology, University of Iowa, 200 Hawkins Drive, Iowa City, IA 52242, USA
[1] Present address: 200 Hawkins Drive, Iowa City, IA 52242.
* Corresponding author. 200 Hawkins Drive, Iowa City, IA 52242.
E-mail address: edgarsama@gmail.com

Neuroimag Clin N Am 34 (2024) 225–240
https://doi.org/10.1016/j.nic.2024.01.003
1052-5149/24/© 2024 Elsevier Inc. All rights reserved.

are aspect ratio (AR) and size ratio (SR). AR measures the degree of elongation of an aneurysm by dividing its perpendicular height by the aneurysm neck.[4] SR, on the other hand, compares the aneurysm's maximal height to the diameter of the parent vessel.[5] A meta-analysis showed that both AR and SR are significantly higher in RIAs compared to UIAs, suggesting that AR and SR may be used as biomarkers of the risk of rupture.[3] However, the heterogeneity of thresholds in determining AR and SR has limited the widespread adoption of these metrics. Additionally, other morphologic characteristics, such as the presence of daughter sacs and irregular lobules, have been associated with an increased risk of rupture,[6] especially in small aneurysms.[6] It is important to note that not all irregularities can be accurately visualized using standard imaging techniques like magnetic resonance angiography (MRA),[7] which may result in some irregularities being missed.

In addition to morphologic evaluation, clinical assessment scales like the PHASES (population, hypertension, age, size of aneurysm, earlier subarachnoid hemorrhage, and site) score have been incorporated into the assessment of UIAs. The PHASES score, derived from a pooled analysis of 6 studies examining the natural course of UIAs, provides a 5-year risk of rupture score. It takes into account various factors such as the patient's descent, age, presence of hypertension, prior aneurysmal subarachnoid hemorrhage (aSAH), and aneurysm size.[8] However, several retrospective studies have not shown an association between ruptured presentation and high PHASES score. In a study of 100 RIAs, approximately 70% of the aneurysms had a 5-year risk of rupture below 2% based on PHASES.[9] The low accuracy of PHASES and other clinical scales have curtailed their use in clinical practice.

Given the limitations of current methods, there has been a growing emphasis on the analysis of the aneurysm wall to identify potential biomarkers of risk of rupture.[10] The aneurysm wall undergoes complex biological processes that may explain aneurysm etiology, growth, and potential rupture.

ANEURYSM WALL COMPOSITION

The aneurysm wall is a complex and dynamic structure that undergoes significant changes during the development and progression of the aneurysm. Histologic studies have provided valuable insights into the characteristics of the aneurysm wall in both RIAs and UIAs (Table 1). Initially, during the formation of an aneurysm, there is a uniform layer of smooth muscle cells lining the luminal surface. However, due to ongoing

hemodynamic stress and the uneven distribution of shear forces, the aneurysm wall becomes heterogeneous.[10] This heterogeneity is characterized by variations in wall thickness and composition.[10,11] Suzuki and colleagues[12] reported a histologic analysis of 23 UIAs with an aneurysm wall thickness that ranged from 0.03 to 0.55 mm. Another study by Acosta and colleagues[13] analyzed 55 aneurysms and reported an average wall thickness of 0.37 ± 0.23 mm. Advanced imaging techniques have revealed that the thickness of the arterial wall can vary significantly within the same aneurysm. In fact, a study by Liu and colleagues[14] analyzed 29 aneurysms and reported variations of up to 3.6 times in wall thickness measurements within a single aneurysm.

Advanced imaging of the arterial wall has been validated with histologic ex-vivo samples. A study of 44 histologic samples obtained from the circle of Willis showed that areas of focal arterial wall thickening on ultrahigh-resolution 7T MR imaging corresponded with advanced atherosclerotic lesions. Signal heterogeneities on 7T MR imaging enabled the spatial differentiation of different plaque components, like foamy macrophages and collagen.[15] Gade and colleagues[16] studied specimens from 17 RIAs and observed calcifications in 11/17 (65%) of cases. Arteriosclerotic changes and intramural hemorrhage were reported in the histologic study of RIAs by Kataoka and colleagues[11] in their analysis of 44 RIAs. Thicker vessel walls may also indicate inflammatory changes and neovascularization.[10] In a study by Liu and colleagues[14] examining a 7-mm anterior communicating artery aneurysm, the thickness of the wall within the aneurysm varied from 0.22 to 0.84 mm. Immunohistochemical analysis demonstrated an abundance of vasa vasorum (small blood vessels that supply the vessel wall) at the thickened part of the aneurysm wall. Furthermore, Kataoka and colleagues[11] confirmed that ruptured and unruptured aneurysms differ in their structural pathology; ruptured aneurysms had a defective endothelium of the inner surface, and their walls tended to be replaced by a hyalinelike structure. Moreover, the walls of RIAs were heterogeneous and were infiltrated by leukocytes. Finally, confocal imaging of specimens from ruptured aneurysms showed the presence of CD8+CD161+ cells within the vessel wall, suggesting an involvement of these immune cells in the pathophysiology of ruptured aneurysms.[17]

IMAGING OF BRAIN ANEURYSMS

There are multiple modalities available to diagnose and monitor intracranial brain aneurysms.

Table 1
Histologic correlates with aneurysm vessel wall imaging

Authors	Sample	Method	Finding
Chyatte et al,[96]	23 UIAs 2 RIAs[a] 11 controls	Immunohistochemistry of aneurysm tissue from patients.	Deposits of complement, IgG, IgM, macrophages, and T lymphocytes were present in the wall of most UIAs but not control arteries
Kataoka et al,[73]	27 UIAs 44 RIAs	Electron microscopy and immunohistochemistry of aneurysm tissue from patients.	RIAs exhibited significant endothelial damage, structural changes of the wall, and inflammatory cell invasion, in contrast to UIAs
Frösen et al,[74]	24 UIAs 42 RIAs	Immunohistochemistry of aneurysm tissue from patients.	RIAs are characterized by apoptosis, de-endothelialization, luminal thrombosis, smooth muscle cell proliferation, and infiltration of T cells and macrophages. Macrophage infiltration was associated with smooth muscle cell proliferation.
Aoki et al.[75]	7 UIAs[b]	Immunohistochemistry and Western blotting of aneurysm in rat model.	MCP-1, a major chemoattractant for monocytes/macrophages, plays a crucial role in the formation and progression of cerebral aneurysms.
Shimonaga et al.[36]	9 UIAs	HR-MR imaging and histopathology of aneurysm tissue from patients.	Wall thickening with the presence of atherosclerosis, neovascularization, and infiltration of inflammatory cells are associated with AWE.
Larsen et al.[76]	13 UIAs	HR-MR imaging and histopathology of aneurysm tissue from patients.	AWE may detect inflammatory and degenerative changes associated with aneurysm progression.

Abbreviations: AWE, aneurysmal wall enhancement; HR, high-resolution; Ig, immunoglobulin; MCP-1, monocyte chemo-attractant protein-1; RIAs, ruptured intracranial aneurysms; UIAs, unruptured intracranial aneurysms.
[a] 11 basilar arteries were used as controls.
[b] Aneurysms were experimentally induced in animal models.

Commonly used modalities include MRA, digital subtraction angiography (DSA), and computed tomography angiography (CTA). The spatial and temporal resolutions of DSA make it the gold standard to characterize aneurysms and to determine morphologic features such as size and the presence of irregularities. Nonetheless, DSA is an invasive procedure that involves navigating a catheter into the patients' brain vasculature and is rarely used to follow UIAs over time.[18] CTA represents an alternative as it provides a sensitivity of more than 95% in detecting aneurysms smaller than 5 mm in size.[19] However, the use of ionizing radiation limits the number of follow-ups that can be done. MRA is another alternative that does not use radiation. Additionally, the sensitivity of MRA for identifying aneurysms smaller than 5 mm may exceed 95%.[20] However, some patients have contraindications to MR imaging such as claustrophobia or non–MR imaging-compatible implants. Despite its high-resolution, contrast-enhanced MRA and time-of-flight MRA may not identify the presence of small daughter sacs with the same accuracy as 3-dimensional (3D) rotational angiography.[7] Furthermore, MRA may underestimate aneurysm volume up to 8% compared to the gold standard DSA.[7] The major limitation DSA, CTA, and MRA is that these are luminal imaging modalities and do not provide information about the aneurysm wall.

High-resolution MR (HR-MR) imaging has the potential to characterize the aneurysm wall but is not routinely used for screening and follow-up. HR-MR imaging has been used to characterize arterial vasculopathies such as vasculitis, atherosclerosis, and aneurysms.[21–24] Sherif and colleagues[25] compared the 3T MR imaging measurements of wall thickness with the histologic measurements of wall thickness in 13 experimental aneurysms. The overestimation of wall thickness on imaging was minimal, averaging only 0.02 mm above the image resolution threshold. This study suggests that the accuracy and reliability of HR-MR imaging in assessing vessel wall thickness are very high. Several HR-MR imaging protocols have been described,[26–28] and the main principle is to suppress intraluminal blood and extraluminal cerebrospinal fluid (CSF), such that the focus of the image is the aneurysm wall itself using small-sized voxels to accurately visualize and assess the wall. The optimal performance of HR-MR imaging for proper visualization of the aneurysm wall starts at 3T MR imaging field strength systems.[29] Feng and colleagues[30] imaged 24 UIAs with both 3T and 7T MR imaging. The study reported a good correlation (r = 0.63 ± 0.19) between aneurysm wall thickness measurements obtained at 3T and 7T. Nonetheless, aneurysm wall thickness measured at 3T was 15% thicker compared to 7T (0.52 ± 0.07 mm vs 0.45 ± 0.05 mm, $P < .001$). Furthermore, wall sharpness at 7T MR imaging was 57% higher compared to 3T MR imaging. The high signal to noise ratio of 7T MR imaging allows a more detailed characterization of the arterial wall.[18] Pohmann and colleagues[31] imaged 3 human subjects in 3T, 7T and 9.4 T scanners. The signal to noise ratio had a supralinear growth with increasing field strength, as indicated by a factor of 3.10 ± 0.20 from 3T to 7T, and 1.76 ± 0.13 from 7T to 9.4 T. Radojewski and colleagues[32] analyzed 30 patients with suspected incidental aneurysms on 3T MR imaging who underwent 7T MR imaging. In all 30 cases, the differentiation of an aneurysm versus a vascular variant could be achieved. In 20 cases (66%), the initial suspected diagnosis was revised. 7T MR imaging systems, however, are limited to only a few centers and are not used in routine clinical practice.

The estimation of wall thickness performed with HR-MR imaging could be very close to its histologic correlate. Sherif and colleagues[33] analyzed 13 bifurcation aneurysms in rabbits. 3T HR-MR imaging with a resolution of 0.4 x 0.4 × 1.5 mm³ was perfomed. Measurements of aneurysm wall thickness performed at the dome were similar to the histologic samples: 0.24 ± 0.06 mm versus 0.30 ± 0.068 mm for HR-MR imaging, $P=.0078$. Similar correlations were reported for measurements performed at the neck: 0.25 ± 0.07 mm versus 0.29 ± 0.07 mm for HR-MR imaging, $P=.0469$. Therefore, vessel wall thickness can be assessed qualitatively by experienced neuroradiologists.[34]

IMAGING OF IRON WITHIN THE ANEURYSM WALL

Ferumoxytol is an iron nanoparticle member of a group known as ultrasmall superparamagnetic iron oxide. It is a promising biomarker for macrophage activity in the arterial wall, as it is phagocyted and cleared by macrophages, and therefore may indirectly be used as a biomarker of inflammation.[35] Hasan and colleagues[36] reported the presence of macrophages within the aneurysm wall using ferumoxytol-enhanced MR imaging. Aneurysms were imaged 24 and 72 hours after ferumoxytol infusion, followed by histologic analysis of the specimens. UIAs with early uptake of ferumoxytol exhibited similar expression levels of various inflammation markers seen in RIAs, including cyclooxygenase-2 and microsomal prostaglandin E2 synthase-1. Furthermore, the expression of these inflammatory molecules was significantly higher in aneurysms with early uptake of ferumoxytol compared to aneurysms with late uptake. All the patients with early aneurysm uptake of ferumoxytol subsequently ruptured.[37] Although the use of ferumoxytol lost momentum due to a black box warning,[38] the in vivo imaging of active macrophages in the aneurysm wall demonstrated that inflammation is at the cornerstone of aneurysm wall biology.

MR imaging sequences have been used to visualize iron and to quantify tissue susceptibility.[39] While susceptibility-weighted images rely on contrast derived from both magnitude and filtered phase images, quantitative susceptibility mapping (QSM) offers the distinct advantage of enabling a quantitative exploration of local tissue susceptibility. This approach also facilitates the differentiation of hypointense calcifications, characterized by their diamagnetic properties, from the hyperintense paramagnetic signals associated with hemorrhagic products.[40] QSM not only provides a direct visualization of susceptibility changes within blood clots but also exhibits the capability to distinguish between acute and chronic hemorrhages.[41] Recent research has further demonstrated the potential of QSM in detecting even subtle hemorrhages within carotid plaques, thereby offering a valuable tool for assessing the vulnerability of atherosclerotic plaques.[42] Collectively, these studies underscore the reliability of QSM as an effective method for detecting the presence of microhemorrhages. The authors' group has used QSM to detect microhemorrhages within the aneurysm wall.[43–45] Forty patients with 51 aneurysms were imaged prospectively with 3T HR-MR imaging and QSM. Microhemorrhages evident on the QSM sequence were detected in 12 (23.5%) intracranial aneurysms (IAs) of 11 subjects. All these subjects had a history of severe headache suggestive of sentinel headache.[46] However, QSM acquisition and processing may be limited by bone artifact. In approximately 30% of cases, microhemorrhages may not be apparent in QSM imaging due imaging artifacts.

ANEURYSMAL WALL ENHANCEMENT

Matouk and colleagues[47] imaged 5 patients with aSAH with HR-MR imaging. The ruptured aneurysms in all cases exhibited aneurysm wall enhancement (AWE), suggesting the presence of active inflammation. Interestingly, among the 3 patients in the case series who had multiple IAs, only the aneurysm that ruptured showed marked enhancement of the vessel wall. In contrast, the other UIAs did not display AWE. Several other studies have reported an association between increased AWE and higher risk of rupture presentation. Three meta-analyses have concluded that AWE is associated with aneurysm instability.[48–50] By providing a detailed visualization of the aneurysm wall, the quantification of AWE through HR-MR imaging could potentially lead to a better understanding of the biological processes that lead to aneurysm formation and rupture.

There are several postulated causes of AWE after the intravenous administration of gadolinium (Gd). First, hemodynamic stress within the aneurysm, such as turbulent blood flow and shear forces, can impact wall enhancement. Hemodynamic patterns inside the aneurysm sac can alter the wall. Disturbed flow patterns and areas of varying wall shear stress (WSS) may trigger inflammatory responses and endothelial dysfunction, leading to increased permeability of the aneurysm wall. These hemodynamic factors can contribute to the development of AWE.[51,52] These processes may be more pronounced in larger aneurysms and lead to higher enhancement. Zhong and colleagues[53] studied 113 anterior circulation UIAs to determine which aneurysm features were associated with AWE. In the multivariate analysis, aneurysm size was the most relevant morphologic feature associated with enhancement.

Second, the location of the aneurysm can also impact AWE. Aneurysms in high-risk locations such as the anterior communicating, posterior communicating, and basilar arteries may exhibit more AWE. A study of 35 aneurysms showed that focal AWE determined by 3D color mapping was higher in aneurysms located in high-risk locations. This finding was consistent for smaller aneurysms as well (<7 mm in diameter).[22]

Third, inflammation in the aneurysm wall may be closely associated with AWE. Inflammatory processes include infiltration of immune cells, release of cytokines, and angiogenesis within the aneurysm wall. These inflammatory responses can lead to vascular remodeling, thinning of the wall, and increased permeability, which may manifest as AWE.[54,55] Inflammation may also lead to thicker walls. Shimonaga and colleagues[54] correlated the histologic findings of 6 aneurysms with HR-MR imaging and reported that most aneurysms with AWE also had wall thickening. Moreover, all of the aneurysms with AWE and wall thickening were positive for the macrophage marker CD68 and the endothelial cell marker CD31. These aneurysms likely had macrophage infiltration and vasa vasorum proliferation.[54] Similarly, Hudson and colleagues[56] analyzed 10 aneurysms and reported that the aneurysms that had a higher AWE also had thicker walls and an increased macrophage infiltration compared to aneurysms without AWE.

Fourth, vascular remodeling appears to be pivotal for AWE. A notable difference between the intracranial and extracranial arteries is that the intracranial arteries do not have vasa vasorum at birth.[57] However, intracranial arteries may develop vasa vasorum in response to disease due to the neovascularization. A histologic study of 50 intracranial arteries observed that vasa vasorum was present in only 36/50 patients. Vasa vasorum seems to be more common in aged patients with severe atherosclerosis and other cerebrovascular diseases.[58] Iihara and colleagues[59] described a case of a giant aneurysm of the vertebral artery that was surrounded by a hyperintense rim after the administration of contrast Gd. On direct observation during surgery, a highly vascularized area of vasa vasorum was observed surrounding the aneurysm. Furthermore, a plexus of small arterioles that may correspond to vasa vasorum and hemosiderin-laden macrophages near the capillaries was observed. Another histologic study by Zhong and colleagues[60] analyzed 41 UIAs and found that inflammatory cell infiltration, intraluminal thrombus, and vasa vasorum were significantly associated with AWE. The presence of vasa vasorum seems to play a role in aneurysm enlargement. A recent study noted vasa vasorum in 25 specimens of IAs in a range of sizes from 3 to 27 mm associated with increased inflammatory infiltrate and intimal hyperplasia.[61]

Finally, AWE may be the result of flow artifact within the aneurysm. Cornelissen and colleagues[62] used a phantom model to simulate aneurysm flow conditions. Near-wall slow flow mimicked AWE. Another study of 6 patients with 14 aneurysms also reported that in 60% of cases, enhancement was at least partially caused by slow intra-aneurysmal flow, leading to pseudo-enhancement of the aneurysm wall.[63] Fortunately, technical advancements of HR-MR imaging may help to avoid this artifact.[34] Black-blood techniques, such as delay alternating with nutation for tailored excitation, have been reported to suppress the signal from the slowly flowing blood.[64] Motion-sensitized driven equilibrium protocols can also be implemented to decrease slow-flow contamination.[65] We also have noticed this phenomenon in HR-MR imaging obtained with 3T and 7T scanners. The visualization of intraluminal "haziness" in T1 and T1-post Gd images is a sign of possible slow-flow artifact.[66]

ANEURYSMAL WALL ENHANCEMENT IN CLINICAL PRACTICE
Can Aneurysmal Wall Enhancement Be Quantified?

AWE is commonly quantified subjectively based on expert consensus. However, this subjective approach may overlook enhancing aneurysms that are not clearly evident and may also include enhancement from other nearby structures such as sinuses and CSF. Furthermore, subjective quantification can be influenced by operator-windowing and field of view. To address these limitations, various objective methods have been proposed for quantifying AWE. One approach involves measuring the signal intensity (SI) of the aneurysmal wall from a 2-dimensional (2D) multiplanar view and obtaining a ratio by dividing this SI to the SI of reference structures such as the corpus callosum, pituitary stalk, and CSF.[67] The objective quantification of AWE aims at providing more reliable and standardized measurements, reducing subjectivity and inter-reader variability. Various quantitative enhancement metrics have been described: (1) aneurysm enhancement ratio $[(SI_{Max}-SI_{pre})/SI_{pre}]$;[68] (2) aneurysm to pituitary stalk contrast ratio $(SI_{wallT1+Gd}/SI_{pituitary\ stalkT1+Gd})$[69]; and (3) aneurysm enhancement index $[(SI_{wallT1+Gd}/SI_{brainT1+Gd})-(SI_{wallT1}/SI_{brainT1})/(SI_{wallT1}/SI_{brainT1})]$.[69] Roa and colleagues[70] investigated 102 UIAs using 3T HR-MR imaging. The mean and maximal SI of the aneurysm wall, the pituitary stalk, and the corpus callosum were quantified on 2D views. These SI values were then compared with different methods of quantifying enhancement, including enhancement ratio, pituitary stalk ratio, and aneurysm enhancement index. The pituitary stalk ratio obtained with the maximal SI values was the most effective method in quantifying enhancement of UIAs.

A potential limitation in quantifying SI is the variability that may exist among scanners from different manufacturers. To address this issue, Roa and colleagues[71] compared the normalized SI measurements of 9 IAs using the same HR-MR imaging protocol. The same subjects underwent a scan in a 3T General Electric and a 3T Siemens scanner. A significant correlation between scanners was reported after normalization to the pituitary stalk (Pearson coefficient = 0.975).

Aneurysms are complex structures that can exhibit irregularities and multiple lobules, which may not be fully captured in 2D views. To overcome this limitation, 3D mapping techniques of AWE have been developed to provide a more comprehensive evaluation of the aneurysmal wall (Fig. 1).[72] SI heat maps may be used to analyze the aneurysm wall of saccular and fusiform aneurysms.[73] The authors' group described a pipeline with various metrics of AWE based on 3D mapping of the aneurysm wall including circumferential, specific, and focal AWE.[67] General AWE quantifies the degree of enhancement in the aneurysm wall normalized to a reference structure, typically the corpus callosum. This measurement provides information on the overall extent of Gd-enhancement along the circumference of the aneurysm wall, enabling comparisons among different aneurysms. Focal AWE reflects specific areas of high enhancement within the aneurysm wall. By defining regions of AWE that are 2 standard deviations above the mean SI of the T1+Gd of the entire aneurysm, we can pinpoint localized areas of heightened enhancement (area $\geq 2\ \sigma$ of T1+Gd$_\mu$). This metric identifies regions of particular interest or potential pathology within the aneurysm, such as blebs. Finally, specific AWE compares the difference on SI before and after the administration of Gd. By assessing the difference between the T1+Gd and pre-contrast T1 imaging, we can determine how much Gd is absorbed within the aneurysm wall (T1+Gdμ $\geq$ T1 μ + 2σ).[67] The information generated through 3D heatmaps can be plotted in histograms for detailed analysis of the distribution of enhancement within the aneurysm wall.[73–75]

How Can Aneurysmal Wall Enhancement Be Used in Clinical Practice?

The assessment of AWE has gained attention as a potential tool for aneurysm risk stratification (Table 2). Omodaka and colleagues[69] studied AWE in 28 RIAs and 76 UIAs. The AWE index was higher

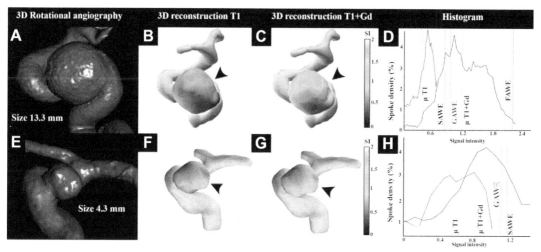

Fig. 1. 3-Dimensional aneurysm wall enhancement (3D-AWE) mapping and histogram analysis of unruptured brain aneurysms. (A) A large internal carotid artery aneurysm of 13.3 mm in diameter had avid enhancement. The 3D-AWE maps before and after gadolinium (Gd) contrast administration (B, C) increased AWE throughout the aneurysm. Notably, specific areas within the aneurysm exhibit even higher levels of AWE (arrowhead). (D) Histogram analysis demonstrates a shift to the right of signal intensity from the pre-Gd curve (black) to the post-Gd curve (red). Specific AWE, general AWE, and focal AWE suggest avid caption of Gd within the wall. Focal AWE is represented as an area within the curve localized beyond 2 standard deviations from the mean T1+Gd value. (E) In contrast, a small internal carotid artery (ICA) aneurysm that measured 4.3 mm in diameter displays mild AWE compared to the larger aneurysm. (F, G) The pre-Gd and post-Gd color maps do not show a significant change in AWE (arrowheads). (H) The histogram also corroborates this lack of enhancement with superimposition of both pre-Gd (black) and post-Gd (red) curves. Notice that the scale in the X axis of the histogram in the non-enhancing aneurysm is lower than the scale for the enhancing aneurysm.

in RIAs than in UIAs. The receiver operating characteristic curve analysis found that a cutoff of 0.53 distinguished RIAs and UIAs with a sensitivity of 96% and a specificity 47%. In a study by Edjlali and colleagues[76] involving 333 UIAs, the investigators defined stable aneurysms as those that were found incidentally and did not change in size over a 6-month period. Conversely, unstable aneurysms were classified as symptomatic or showing changes in size over the same duration. Enhancement was graded as grade 0 for none or questionable focal trace enhancement, grade 1 for focal thick (>1 mm) enhancement, grade 2 for thin (maximum thickness, ≤1 mm) circumferential AWE, or grade 3 for thick (maximum thickness, >1 mm) circumferential AWE. Grade 3 enhancement demonstrated the highest specificity (84.4%) and negative predictive value (94.3%) for distinguishing between stable and unstable aneurysms.[76] In a study by Nagahata and colleagues[77] comparing 83 RIAs and 61 UIAs, strong and faint AWE were present in 73.8% and 24.6% of the RIAs, respectively, and in 4.8% and 13.3% of the UIAs. Approximately 81.9% of the UIAs showed no enhancement. Wang and colleagues[78] studied a total of 19 RIAs and 72 UIAs. RIAs had enhancement ratio higher than UIAs (odds ratio [OR] 6.64, 95% confidence interval [CI] 1.91–22.97).

Raghuram and colleagues[67] performed 3D AWE mapping of a cohort of 33 UIAs using 7T HR-MR imaging and determined that general aneurysm wall enhancement was higher in aneurysms with a size ≥ 7 mm. Moreover, blebs had higher enhancement than the rest of the aneurysm body.

AWE may also be useful in determining the risk of aneurysm growth. Gariel and colleagues[79] evaluated 145 UIAs using 3T HR-MR imaging. A total of 12 (8.3%) aneurysms displayed morphologic growth at the 2-year follow-up. In their multivariable analysis, increased AWE was associated with UIA growth (relative risk 26.1, 95% CI, 7.4–91.7, P<.001). Increased AWE during follow-up also had a positive predictive value of 96% and a negative predictive value of 100% for growth. AWE may also be used to identify which aneurysms may change in morphology. Matsushige and colleagues[80] analyzed 60 aneurysms at baseline and follow-up using HR-MR imaging. Based on the UIAs' behavior, aneurysms were labeled as stable, whole sac expansion, or daughter sac formation. AWE was less frequently observed in stable UIAs compared to UIAs that underwent morphologic changes at follow-up. Also, aneurysms with daughter sac formation showed a significantly higher frequency of AWE than those that only had whole sac expansion. Omodaka

Table 2
Aneurysmal wall enhancement studies

Authors	Outcome	Sample	Quantification	AWE	SN	SP
Nagahata et al,[77] 2016	Rupture	61 RIAs 83 UIAs	Qualitative	Strong, faint AWE and no AWE[a]	73.8%	94.2%
Wang et al,[78] 2018	Rupture	19 RIAs 87 UIAs	Objective 2D	Enhancement ratio[b] (cutoff value 61.5%)	89.5%	63.2%
Omodaka et al,[69] 2016	Rupture	28 RIAs 76 UIAs	Objective 2D	Wall enhancement index (cutoff value 0.53)[c]	96%	47%
Matsushige et al,[80] 2019	Morphologic change	60 UIAs	Qualitative	Presence or Absence	72%	72%
Omodaka et al,[81] 2019	Evolution[d]	26 evolving, 69 stable, and 67 ruptured	Objective 2D	CRstalk (cutoff value 0.39)	88%	63%
Gariel et al,[79] 2020	Growth	145 UIAs	Qualitative	De novo or increase in intensity, extension, or thickness of AWE	83%	58%
Edjlali et al,[76] 2018	Symptomatic and morphologic change	307 UIAs: 276 stable[e], 31 unstable; 26 RIAs	Qualitative	0: none, 1: focal, 2: thin circumferential, 3: thick (>1 mm) circumferential	70.9%	61.6%
Wang et al,[97] 2019	Symptomatic onset	89 UIAs	Objective 2D	Enhancement ratio (cutoff 60.5%)	90.3%	87.9%
Raghuram et al,[22] 2022	Symptomatic onset	88 UIAs 5 RIAs	Objective 3D-AWE maps	3D circumferential AWE, specific AWE, focal AWE	80%[f]	90%
Fu et al,[82] 2021	Symptomatic onset	341 UIAs	Qualitative Objective 2D	No/focal/circumferential; Wall enhancement index	95.7%	73.4%
Roa et al,[70] 2020	Size>7 mm	102 UIAs	Objective 2D	CRstalk (cutoff value 0.60)	81.5%	61%

Abbreviations: AWE, aneurysmal wall enhancement; CRstalk, contrast ratio of the aneurysm wall against the pituitary stalk; ER, enhancement ratio; RIA, ruptured intracranial aneurysm; SI, signal intensity; SN, sensitivity; SP, specificity; UIA, unruptured intracranial aneurysm.

a "Strong enhancement" was defined as definite enhancement equal to choroid plexus or venous plexus. "Faint enhancement" was defined as increased wall signal intensity than precontrast scan. Sensitivity and specificity values are reported for the presence of 'strong enhancement.'

b Enhancement ratio: (SImax − SIpre)/SIpre × 100%.

c Wall enhancement index: ((SIwall/SIbrain on postcontrast imaging] − [SIwall/SIbrain on matched precontrast imaging])/(SIwall/SIbrain on matched precontrast imaging).

d Aneurysm evolution defined as growth and symptomatic onset. CRstalk: SIwall/SIstalk.

e "Stable was defined as no morphologic changes, "whole sac expansion" was defined as enlargement of the whole aneurysm sac, and "daughter sac formation" was defined as development of a bleb or another aneurysmal component. Sensitivity reported for no AWE versus any AWE.

f Sensitivity and specificity are reported for a model that included 3D circumferential AWE+, age, female gender, and focal AWE.

and colleagues[81] compared 26 evolving aneurysms to 69 stable aneurysms and 67 RIAs. The investigators defined an aneurysm as evolving if it presented symptoms or had growth at follow-up. The AWE normalized to the pituitary stalk ratio in evolving aneurysms was significantly higher than in stable aneurysms (0.54 vs 0.34) and lower than RIAs (0.54 vs 0.83). A pituitary stalk ratio of 0.39 had a 0.88 sensitivity and a 0.63 specificity for detecting evolving aneurysm.

AWE may correlate with the presentation of UIAs. Fu and colleagues[82] studied 341 UIAs of which 93 were symptomatic and 248 were asymptomatic. Circumferential AWE was more common in symptomatic than asymptomatic UIAs (66.7% vs 17.3%). In the multivariate analysis, both the AWE pattern and the AWE index were independent factors associated with symptomatic status (AWE index OR 3.32). Both the AWE pattern and the AWE index had an area under the curve (AUC) of 0.91 for identifying symptomatic UIAs, with a sensitivity of 95.7% and a specificity of 73.4%. The authors' group used the 3D AWE mapping pipeline in the analysis of 93 saccular aneurysms that were imaged using 3T HR-MR imaging. Symptomatic aneurysms were defined as ruptured, or if they presented with sentinel headache or cranial nerve neuropathy.[75] Circumferential AWE, specific AWE, and focal AWE were all associated with symptomatic status (OR = 1.34, 1.25, and 1.08, respectively). The authors generated a multivariate logistic regression model that included aneurysm size, circumferential AWE, histogram skewness, age, and female gender. This model detected symptomatic status with 80% specificity and 90% sensitivity. Focal AWE was significantly associated with irregular aneurysm morphology.

While AWE is significantly more frequent in symptomatic, unstable, ruptured, or growing aneurysms as compared to stable UIAs, it may also be seen in stable UIAs. A meta-analysis performed by Texakalidis and colleagues[49] found that the lack of AWE was a strong predictor for aneurysm stability. More than 90% of saccular aneurysms without circumferential AWE remain unruptured and asymptomatic. The authors use the lack of AWE in their clinical practice in determining which aneurysm ruptured when patients with aSAH present with multiple aneurysms. In instances when it is impossible to determine which aneurysm ruptured based on morphologic features of blood distribution in the subarachnoid space, the authors used the lack of AWE to determine which aneurysm did not rupture.

AWE can also be used to monitor UIAs that are treated medically. A recent randomized controlled trial that involved the longitudinal imaging of UIAs, with baseline AWE measurements, reported that patients who were treated with atorvastatin had decreased AWE at the 6-month follow-up ($P < .01$).[83] Conversely, the placebo group showed no significant decline in AWE ($P = .27$). Notably, alterations in serum inflammatory markers such as interleukin 6, C-reactive protein, and tumor necrosis factor α, mirrored the shifts in AWE. Remarkably, no discernible changes surfaced in aneurysm morphology or size, thereby corroborating the notion that AWE on HR-MR imaging holds the potential to surpass aneurysm morphology as a superior marker for gauging treatment response. Edjlali and colleagues[84] also reported a case of a large carotid ophthalmic aneurysm with thick AWE and optic nerve palsy. The patient refused surgical treatment and was treated medically with steroids. On follow-up imaging, the AWE and cranial neuropathy resolved. This observation suggested an anti-inflammatory effect of steroids on AWE that may have contributed to the resolution of the optic nerve palsy.

MULTIMODAL IMAGING OF ANEURYSMS
Aneurysmal Wall Enhancement, Computational Flow Dynamics, and Wall Tension

AWE may be influenced by flow patterns inside the aneurysm.[72] Zhang and colleagues[85] studied 49 UIAs with 4-dimensional flow MR imaging and reported that areas of low WSS, which are caused by low flow conditions, correlated with areas of high AWE. Similarly, Hadad and colleagues[86] imaged 23 aneurysms with 7T HR-MR imaging and determined that areas of the aneurysm with AWE had a lower WSS compared to areas without enhancement. The pattern of AWE, flow conditions, and stresses imposed on the aneurysm wall may vary among the different regions of the aneurysm. The detailed analysis of aneurysm morphomechanics and AWE suggests that the aneurysm neck, body, and dome are exposed to different flow environments. The mechanical stress at the neck is higher than at the dome due to the inflow jet from the parent artery. Areas of AWE at the neck have higher WSS gradients compared to areas without AWE. Contrarily, regions of AWE at the aneurysm body have lower WSS compared to areas that do not have AWE.[86]

The authors' group has developed a post-acquisition imaging pipeline for the coregistration of AWE maps, finite element analysis maps, and computational fluid dynamics (Fig. 2).[87] Twenty-six UIAs were imaged with 7T HR-MR imaging. Areas of AWE in the dome exhibited lower WSS

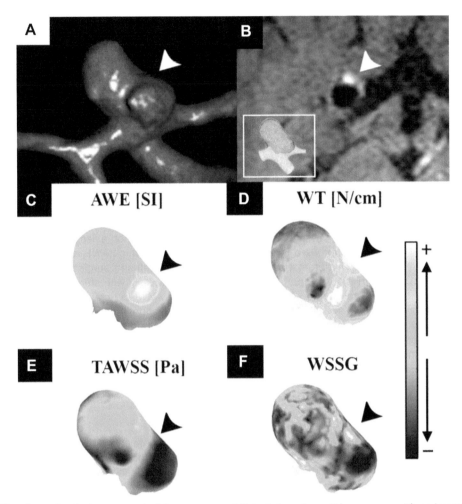

Fig. 2. Morphomechanical assessment of the aneurysm. (A) An internal carotid aneurysm with an irregular small lobule (*arrowhead*) is analyzed with our pipeline for 3-dimensional mapping of aneurysm wall enhancement (AWE), finite element analysis (FEA), and computational fluid dynamics (CFD). (B) The 3 T high-resolution (HR) MR imaging demonstrates a clear area of AWE at the location of the irregular lobule (*arrowhead*). (C) The area of high AWE in the irregular lobule is represented in the 3D color map of the aneurysm (*arrowhead*) as a yellow circular area. The pipeline allows the coregistration with FEA and CFD metrics. (D) Wall tension (WT, *arrowhead*) appears to be high, close to the curvature where the irregular lobule originates. (*E, F*) CFD analysis shows that time average wall shear stress (TAWSS) and wall shear stress gradient (WSSG) are not particularly high at the irregular lobule (*arrowheads*).

than areas located in the neck. Additionally, when compared to areas of the sac without AWE, blebs exhibited higher AWE, lower wall tension, and lower WSS. Conversely, the neck had average AWE, high wall tension, and high WSS consistent with high flow conditions. Larsen and colleagues[88] also reported that focal AWE is colocalized with hemodynamic factors associated with higher rupture risk. In their analysis of 22 aneurysms, regions of the aneurysm with AWE also exhibited low WSS. Histologic analysis showed the presence of inflammation and wall degeneration in areas of focal AWE. Khan and colleagues[89] analyzed 22 aneurysms and also determined that

aneurysms with AWE had lower WSS than the non-AWE group.

Radiomics in Aneurysm Imaging

Radiomics is a novel automatic imaging processing tool for pixel-by-pixel extraction of object features, including voxel intensity–based and shape-based parameters (Fig. 3).[18,90–92] For instance, radiomics features have been utilized to identify aneurysms at risk of rupture and predict incomplete occlusion following flow diversion placement. In a study involving 58 treated aneurysms, 16 shape features calculated through

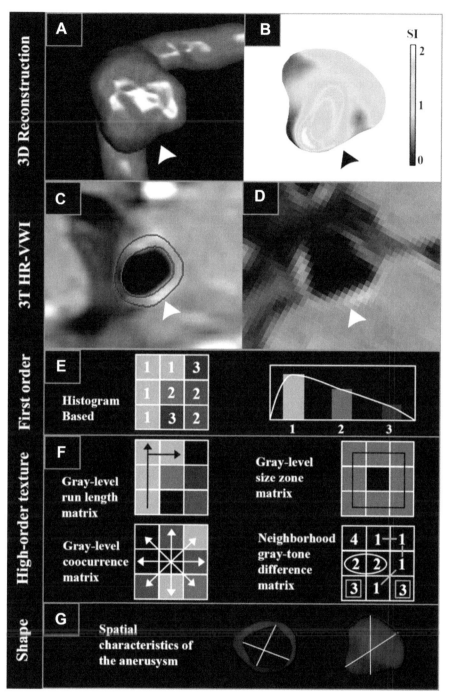

Fig. 3. Radiomics features extraction of the aneurysm wall. (*A*) 3D rotational angiography reconstruction of an irregular distal internal carotid artery aneurysm (*arrowhead*). (*B*) The aneurysm wall can be mapped by generating a 3-dimensional heatmap of signal intensity (SI). In this case, an area of high SI is observed in the irregular area of the aneurysm (*arrowhead*) (*C*) A multiplanar segmentation of the aneurysm wall (*arrowhead*) is obtained, to generate a 3D color map of the aneurysm. This segmentation will then be used to extract radiomic features (*D*). The aneurysm wall includes heterogeneous areas with high enhancement (*arrowhead*) and is comprehensively analyzed with more than 100 radiomics features. (*E*) First-order features include features that are calculated from a histogram-based approach and only measure the frequency of different signal intensities in the image. These include the median value, the standard deviation, kurtosis, and skewness of the histogram. In the first-order radiomics, the organization of SI in space is not considered in the metrics. (*F*) High-order textural features incorporate the localization of SI voxels in space. Gray level co-occurrence matrix measures how frequently a voxel pair occurs in space. Gray-level run length matrix evaluates how many seminal SI voxels occur contiguously. Neighborhood gray-tone difference matrix represents the difference between one voxel and the surrounding voxels. Gray-level size zone matrix evaluates how many voxels with the same value occur contiguously to represent how homogeneous an image is. (*G*) Shape-based radiomics features, such as elongation, maximal diameter, volume, can also be calculated automatically from the segmentation.

radiomics identified predictors of incomplete occlusion, with higher elongation values independently associated with incomplete occlusion.[93] Machine learning has been used to determine which radiomic features are more accurate at detecting unstable aneurysms. Liu and colleagues[94] analyzed 420 aneurysms and defined flatness as the most important morphologic feature to predict aneurysms instability, followed by spherical disproportion, maximum 2D diameter slice, and surface area. Notably, a multivariate model combining AR, SR, and elongation index achieved a higher AUC compared to a model incorporating elongation and flatness (AUC = 0.79 vs AUC = 0.75).[90] Ludwig and colleagues[95] analyzed 353 aneurysms from 3D rotational angiography datasets and extracted 13 radiomic features. Radiomics-derived elongation and flatness were the best predictors of rupture status with AUC values of 0.71 and 0.72, respectively, consistent with the results from Liu and colleagues.[94] However, several established parameters, such as AR (AUC = 0.75), non-sphericity index (AUC = 0.75), height/width (AUC = 0.73), and SR (AUC = 0.73), outperformed radiomics for rupture status discrimination. Radiomics demonstrates great promise in the analysis of the arterial wall, offering a comprehensive and in-depth assessment of SI. The authors' group analyzed 126 aneurysms and found 75 radiomic features that were significantly different between high-risk and low-risk aneurysms.[92] The radiomics model achieved a 90% accuracy in detecting high-risk aneurysms. Risk was determined based on a PHASES score $\geq$ 6. The ability of radiomics to generate, in an automated fashion, a large amount of texture-derived features from a variety of image modalities makes it an attractive tool for machine learning and medical informatics research.

SUMMARY

The imaging of the aneurysm wall with HR-MR imaging has the potential to advance our understanding of aneurysm biology. The evaluation of AWE can potentially be used for risk stratification and monitoring of aneurysm progression. By combining AWE assessment with established risk factors, such as aneurysm size, location, and patient-specific characteristics, a more comprehensive evaluation of aneurysm rupture risk can be achieved. Furthermore, emerging modalities of analysis that incorporate flow and wall tension metrics may generate a more comprehensive assessment. Machine learning and radiomics have the potential to determine high-risk characteristics through the analysis of large datasets.

CLINICS CARE POINTS

- The current approach to triaging aneurysms for treatment or radiological monitoring relies solely on clinical scales, which only account for size in the morphologic assessment of aneurysms.
- In the authors' proposal, the authors advocate for a comprehensive evaluation that encompasses not only size but also factors like shape, the identification of irregularities, and the assessment of Gd enhancement in the aneurysm wall. This multifaceted approach aims to enhance the accuracy of risk assessment for aneurysm rupture.
- Certain studies propose that in cases where distinguishing the ruptured aneurysm is challenging among patients with aSAH and with multiple aneurysms, the aneurysm exhibiting a higher degree of wall enhancement could potentially identify the aneurysm that has ruptured.

FUNDING

Grants from the Brain Anerysm Foundation and the Bee Foundation.

DISCLOSURE

The authors have nothing to disclose.

REFERENCES

1. Wiebers DO, Whisnant JP, Huston J 3rd, et al. Unruptured intracranial aneurysms: natural history, clinical outcome, and risks of surgical and endovascular treatment. Lancet 2003;362(9378):103–10.
2. Waqas M, Chin F, Rajabzadeh-Oghaz H, et al. Size of ruptured intracranial aneurysms: a systematic review and meta-analysis. Acta Neurochir 2020; 162(6):1353–62.
3. Sanchez S., Hickerson M., Patel R.R., et al., Morphological Characteristics of Ruptured Brain Aneurysms: A Systematic Literature Review and Meta-Analysis. Stroke: Vascular and Interventional Neurology. 2023, 0(0):e000707.
4. Ujiie H, Tamano Y, Sasaki K, et al. Is the aspect ratio a reliable index for predicting the rupture of a saccular aneurysm? Neurosurgery 2001;48(3): 495–502 [discussion: 502–3].
5. Dhar S, Tremmel M, Mocco J, et al. Morphology parameters for intracranial aneurysm rupture risk assessment. Neurosurgery 2008;63(2):185–96 [discussion: 196–7].

6. Lindgren AE, Koivisto T, Björkman J, et al. Irregular Shape of Intracranial Aneurysm Indicates Rupture Risk Irrespective of Size in a Population-Based Cohort. Stroke 2016;47(5):1219–26.

7. Raghuram A, Patel R, Varon A, et al. Volumetric surveillance of brain aneurysms: Pitfalls of MRA. Interv Neuroradiol 2022. https://doi.org/10.1177/15910199221100619. 15910199221100619.

8. Greving JP, Wermer MJH, Brown RD, et al. Development of the PHASES score for prediction of risk of rupture of intracranial aneurysms: a pooled analysis of six prospective cohort studies. Lancet Neurol 2014;13(1):59–66.

9. Neyazi B, Sandalcioglu IE, Maslehaty H. Evaluation of the risk of rupture of intracranial aneurysms in patients with aneurysmal subarachnoid hemorrhage according to the PHASES score. Neurosurg Rev 2019;42(2):489–92.

10. Samaniego EA. Brain Aneurysm Biology: What Can We Learn From Imaging? Stroke: Vascular and Interventional Neurology 2022;2(6):e000629.

11. Kataoka K, Taneda M, Asai T, et al. Structural Fragility and Inflammatory Response of Ruptured Cerebral Aneurysms. Stroke 1999;30(7):1396–401.

12. Suzuki J, Ohara H. Clinicopathological study of cerebral aneurysms. Origin, rupture, repair, and growth. J Neurosurg 1978;48(4):505–14.

13. Acosta JM, Cayron AF, Dupuy N, et al. Effect of Aneurysm and Patient Characteristics on Intracranial Aneurysm Wall Thickness. Front Cardiovasc Med 2021;8:775307.

14. Liu X, Feng J, Li Z, et al. Quantitative analysis of unruptured intracranial aneurysm wall thickness and enhancement using 7T high resolution, black blood magnetic resonance imaging. J Neurointerventional Surg 2022;14(7):723–8.

15. van der Kolk AG, Zwanenburg JJ, Denswil NP, et al. Imaging the intracranial atherosclerotic vessel wall using 7T MRI: initial comparison with histopathology. AJNR Am J Neuroradiol 2015;36(4):694–701.

16. Gade PS, Tulamo R, Lee K-w, et al. Calcification in Human Intracranial Aneurysms Is Highly Prevalent and Displays Both Atherosclerotic and Nonatherosclerotic Types. Arterioscler Thromb Vasc Biol 2019;39(10):2157–67.

17. Roa JA, Sarkar D, Zanaty M, et al. Preliminary results in the analysis of the immune response after aneurysmal subarachnoid hemorrhage. Sci Rep 2020;10(1):11809.

18. Beaman C, Patel SD, Nael K, et al. Imaging of Intracranial Saccular Aneurysms. Stroke: Vascular and Interventional Neurology. 0(0):e000757.https://doi.org/10.1161/SVIN.122.000757.

19. Yang ZL, Ni QQ, Schoepf UJ, et al. Small Intracranial Aneurysms: Diagnostic Accuracy of CT Angiography. Radiology 2017;285(3):941–52.

20. Li MH, Li YD, Gu BX, et al. Accurate diagnosis of small cerebral aneurysms ≤5 mm in diameter with 3.0-T MR angiography. Radiology 2014;271(2):553–60.

21. Fakih R, Varon Miller A, Raghuram A, et al. High resolution 7T MR imaging in characterizing culprit intracranial atherosclerotic plaques. Intervent Neuroradiol 2022. https://doi.org/10.1177/15910199221145760. 15910199221145760.

22. Raghuram A, Sanchez S, Wendt L, et al. 3D aneurysm wall enhancement is associated with symptomatic presentation. J Neurointerventional Surg 2022. https://doi.org/10.1136/jnis-2022-019125. neurintsurg-2022-019125.

23. Sanchez S, Raghuram A, Fakih R, et al. 3D Enhancement Color Maps in the Characterization of Intracranial Atherosclerotic Plaques. AJNR Am J Neuroradiol 2022;43(9):1252–8.

24. Mandell DM, Matouk CC, Farb RI, et al. Vessel Wall MRI to Differentiate Between Reversible Cerebral Vasoconstriction Syndrome and Central Nervous System Vasculitis. Stroke 2012;43(3):860–2.

25. Sherif C, Kleinpeter G, Mach G, et al. Evaluation of cerebral aneurysm wall thickness in experimental aneurysms: comparison of 3T-MR imaging with direct microscopic measurements. Acta Neurochir 2014;156(1):27–34.

26. Balu N, Zhou Z, Hippe DS, et al. Accelerated multicontrast high isotropic resolution 3D intracranial vessel wall MRI using a tailored k-space undersampling and partially parallel reconstruction strategy. Magma 2019;32(3):343–57.

27. Kalsoum E, Chabernaud Negrier A, Tuilier T, et al. Blood Flow Mimicking Aneurysmal Wall Enhancement: A Diagnostic Pitfall of Vessel Wall MRI Using the Postcontrast 3D Turbo Spin-Echo MR Imaging Sequence. AJNR Am J Neuroradiol 2018;39(6):1065–7.

28. Qiao Y, Steinman DA, Qin Q, et al. Intracranial arterial wall imaging using three-dimensional high isotropic resolution black blood MRI at 3.0 Tesla. J Magn Reson Imaging 2011;34(1):22–30.

29. Lehman VT, Brinjikji W, Mossa-Basha M, et al. Conventional and high-resolution vessel wall MRI of intracranial aneurysms: current concepts and new horizons. J Neurosurg 2018;128(4):969–81.

30. Feng J, Liu X, Zhang Z, et al. Comparison of 7 T and 3 T vessel wall MRI for the evaluation of intracranial aneurysm wall. Eur Radiol 2022;32(4):2384–92.

31. Pohmann R, Speck O, Scheffler K. Signal-to-noise ratio and MR tissue parameters in human brain imaging at 3, 7, and 9.4 tesla using current receive coil arrays. Magn Reson Med 2016;75(2):801–9.

32. Radojewski P, Slotboom J, Joseph A, et al. Clinical Implementation of 7T MRI for the Identification of Incidental Intracranial Aneurysms versus Anatomic Variants. AJNR Am J Neuroradiol 2021;42(12):2172–4.

33. Sherif C, Kleinpeter G, Loyoddin M, et al. Aneurysm wall thickness measurements of experimental aneurysms: in vivo high-field MR imaging versus direct microscopy. Acta Neurochir Suppl 2015;120:17–20.

34. Diab R, Chang D, Zhu C, et al. Advanced cross-sectional imaging of cerebral aneurysms. Br J Radiol 2023;96(1141):20220686.

35. Chalouhi N, Jabbour P, Magnotta V, et al. Molecular imaging of cerebrovascular lesions. Transl Stroke Res 2014;5(2):260–8.

36. Hasan DM, Mahaney KB, Magnotta VA, et al. Macrophage imaging within human cerebral aneurysms wall using ferumoxytol-enhanced MRI: a pilot study. Arterioscler Thromb Vasc Biol 2012;32(4):1032–8.

37. Hasan D, Chalouhi N, Jabbour P, et al. Early Change in Ferumoxytol-Enhanced Magnetic Resonance Imaging Signal Suggests Unstable Human Cerebral Aneurysm. Stroke 2012;43(12):3258–65.

38. Rubin R. Black Box Warning for Anemia Drug. JAMA 2015;313(17):1704.

39. Liu T, Surapaneni K, Lou M, et al. Cerebral microbleeds: burden assessment by using quantitative susceptibility mapping. Radiology 2012;262(1):269–78.

40. Zhang S, Chiang GC, Knapp JM, et al. Grading meningiomas utilizing multiparametric MRI with inclusion of susceptibility weighted imaging and quantitative susceptibility mapping. J Neuroradiol 2020;47(4):272–7.

41. Schneider TM, Nagel AM, Zorn M, et al. Quantitative susceptibility mapping and (23) Na imaging-based in vitro characterization of blood clotting kinetics. NMR Biomed 2018;31(6):e3926.

42. Ikebe Y, Ishimaru H, Imai H, et al. Quantitative Susceptibility Mapping for Carotid Atherosclerotic Plaques: A Pilot Study. Magn Reson Med Sci 2020;19(2):135–40.

43. Nakagawa D, Kudo K, Awe O, et al. Detection of microbleeds associated with sentinel headache using MRI quantitative susceptibility mapping: pilot study. J Neurosurg 2018;130(4):1391–7.

44. Nakagawa D, Cushing C, Nagahama Y, et al. Quantitative Susceptibility Mapping as a Possible Tool to Radiographically Diagnose Sentinel Headache Associated with Intracranial Aneurysm: Case Report. World Neurosurg 2017;103:954 e1–e954 e4.

45. Sabotin RP, Varon A, Roa JA, et al. Insights into the pathogenesis of cerebral fusiform aneurysms: high-resolution MRI and computational analysis. J Neurointerv Surg 2021;13(12):1180–6.

46. Ishii D, Nakagawa D, Zanaty M, et al. Quantitative Susceptibility Mapping and Vessel Wall Imaging as Screening Tools to Detect Microbleed in Sentinel Headache. J Clin Med 2020;9(4). https://doi.org/10.3390/jcm9040979.

47. Matouk CC, Mandell DM, Günel M, et al. Vessel wall magnetic resonance imaging identifies the site of rupture in patients with multiple intracranial aneurysms: proof of principle. Neurosurgery 2013;72(3):492–6 [discussion: 496].

48. Larson AS, Lehman VT, Lanzino G, et al. Lack of Baseline Intracranial Aneurysm Wall Enhancement Predicts Future Stability: A Systematic Review and Meta-Analysis of Longitudinal Studies. AJNR Am J Neuroradiol 2020;41(9):1606–10.

49. Texakalidis P, Hilditch CA, Lehman V, et al. Vessel Wall Imaging of Intracranial Aneurysms: Systematic Review and Meta-analysis. World Neurosurg 2018;117:453–458 e1.

50. Molenberg R, Aalbers MW, Appelman APA, et al. Intracranial aneurysm wall enhancement as an indicator of instability: a systematic review and meta-analysis. Eur J Neurol 2021;28(11):3837–48.

51. Raghuram A, Galloy A, Nino M, et al. Comprehensive morphomechanical analysis of brain aneurysms. Acta Neurochir 2023. https://doi.org/10.1007/s00701-022-05476-4.

52. Lv N, Karmonik C, Chen S, et al. Wall Enhancement, Hemodynamics, and Morphology in Unruptured Intracranial Aneurysms with High Rupture Risk. Transl Stroke Res 2020;11(5):882–9.

53. Zhong W, Du Y, Guo Q, et al. The Clinical and Morphologic Features Related to Aneurysm Wall Enhancement and Enhancement Pattern in Patients with Anterior Circulation Aneurysms. World Neurosurgery 2020;134:e649–56.

54. Shimonaga K, Matsushige T, Ishii D, et al. Clinicopathological Insights From Vessel Wall Imaging of Unruptured Intracranial Aneurysms. Stroke 2018;49(10):2516–9.

55. Edjlali M, Gentric J-C, Régent-Rodriguez C, et al. Does Aneurysmal Wall Enhancement on Vessel Wall MRI Help to Distinguish Stable From Unstable Intracranial Aneurysms? Stroke 2014;45(12):3704–6.

56. Hudson JS, Zanaty M, Nakagawa D, et al. Magnetic Resonance Vessel Wall Imaging in Human Intracranial Aneurysms. Stroke 2018. https://doi.org/10.1161/STROKEAHA.118.023701. STROKEAHA118023701.

57. Aydin F. Do human intracranial arteries lack vasa vasorum? A comparative immunohistochemical study of intracranial and systemic arteries. Acta Neuropathol 1998;96(1):22–8.

58. Takaba M, Endo S, Kurimoto M, et al. Vasa vasorum of the intracranial arteries. Acta Neurochir 1998;140(5):411–6.

59. Iihara K, Murao K, Sakai N, et al. Continued growth of and increased symptoms from a thrombosed giant aneurysm of the vertebral artery after complete endovascular occlusion and trapping: the role of vasa vasorum: Case report. J Neurosurg 2003;98(2):407–13.

60. Zhong W, Su W, Li T, et al. Aneurysm Wall Enhancement in Unruptured Intracranial Aneurysms: A Histopathological Evaluation. J Am Heart Assoc 2021;10(2):e018633.

61. Wen D, Kieran NW, Yu Z, et al. Presence of vasa vasorum in human intracranial aneurysms. Acta Neurochir 2020;162(9):2283–93.

62. Cornelissen BMW, Leemans EL, Coolen BF, et al. Insufficient slow-flow suppression mimicking aneurysm wall enhancement in magnetic resonance vessel wall imaging: a phantom study. Neurosurg Focus 2019;47(1):E19.

63. Cornelissen BMW, Leemans EL, Slump CH, et al. Vessel wall enhancement of intracranial aneurysms: fact or artifact? Neurosurg Focus 2019;47(1):E18.

64. Li L, Miller KL, Jezzard P. DANTE-prepared pulse trains: a novel approach to motion-sensitized and motion-suppressed quantitative magnetic resonance imaging. Magn Reson Med 2012;68(5):1423–38.

65. Pravdivtseva MS, Gaidzik F, Berg P, et al. Pseudo-Enhancement in Intracranial Aneurysms on Black-Blood MRI: Effects of Flow Rate, Spatial Resolution, and Additional Flow Suppression. J Magn Reson Imaging 2021;54(3):888–901.

66. Samaniego EA, Roa JA, Hasan D. Vessel wall imaging in intracranial aneurysms. J Neurointerv Surg 2019. https://doi.org/10.1136/neurintsurg-2019-014938.

67. Raghuram A, Varon A, Roa JA, et al. Semiautomated 3D mapping of aneurysmal wall enhancement with 7T-MRI. Sci Rep 2021;11(1):18344.

68. Wang GX, Wen L, Lei S, et al. Wall enhancement ratio and partial wall enhancement on MRI associated with the rupture of intracranial aneurysms. J Neurointerv Surg 2018;10(6):566–70.

69. Omodaka S, Endo H, Niizuma K, et al. Quantitative Assessment of Circumferential Enhancement along the Wall of Cerebral Aneurysms Using MR Imaging. AJNR Am J Neuroradiol 2016;37(7):1262–6.

70. Roa JA, Fakih R, Zanaty M, et al. Quantitative Assessment of Ventriculostomy-Related Hemorrhage: A Volume-Based Classification System to Predict New Neurological Symptoms. Oper Neurosurg (Hagerstown) 2020. https://doi.org/10.1093/ons/opaa319.

71. Roa JA, Zanaty M, Osorno-Cruz C, et al. Objective quantification of contrast enhancement of unruptured intracranial aneurysms: a high-resolution vessel wall imaging validation study. J Neurosurg 2020. https://doi.org/10.3171/2019.12.JNS192746.

72. Veeturi SS, Rajabzadeh-Oghaz H, Pintér NK, et al. Aneurysm risk metrics and hemodynamics are associated with greater vessel wall enhancement in intracranial aneurysms. R Soc Open Sci 2021;8(11):211119.

73. Raghuram A, Varon A, Sanchez S, et al. Topographical Analysis of Aneurysm Wall Enhancement With 3-Dimensional Mapping. Stroke Vasc Interv Neurol 2022;2(4). https://doi.org/10.1161/svin.121.000309.

74. Raghuram A, Varon A, Roa JA, et al. Semiautomated 3D mapping of aneurysmal wall enhancement with 7T-MRI. Sci Rep-Uk 2021;11(1). ARTN 18344.

75. Raghuram A, Sanchez S, Wendt L, et al. 3D aneurysm wall enhancement is associated with symptomatic presentation. J Neurointerv Surg. 2022;doi:10.1136/jnis-2022-019125.

76. Edjlali M, Guédon A, Hassen WB, et al. Circumferential Thick Enhancement at Vessel Wall MRI Has High Specificity for Intracranial Aneurysm Instability. Radiology 2018;289(1):181–7.

77. Nagahata S, Nagahata M, Obara M, et al. Wall Enhancement of the Intracranial Aneurysms Revealed by Magnetic Resonance Vessel Wall Imaging Using Three-Dimensional Turbo Spin-Echo Sequence with Motion-Sensitized Driven-Equilibrium: A Sign of Ruptured Aneurysm? Clin Neuroradiol 2016;26(3):277–83.

78. Wang G-x, Wen L, Lei S, et al. Wall enhancement ratio and partial wall enhancement on MRI associated with the rupture of intracranial aneurysms. J Neurointerventional Surg 2018;10(6):566–70.

79. Gariel F, Ben Hassen W, Boulouis G, et al. Increased Wall Enhancement During Follow-Up as a Predictor of Subsequent Aneurysmal Growth. Stroke 2020;51(6):1868–72.

80. Matsushige T, Shimonaga K, Ishii D, et al. Vessel Wall Imaging of Evolving Unruptured Intracranial Aneurysms. Stroke 2019;50(7):1891–4.

81. Omodaka S, Endo H, Niizuma K, et al. Circumferential wall enhancement in evolving intracranial aneurysms on magnetic resonance vessel wall imaging. Journal of Neurosurgery JNS 2019;131(4):1262–8.

82. Fu Q, Wang Y, Zhang Y, et al. Qualitative and Quantitative Wall Enhancement on Magnetic Resonance Imaging Is Associated With Symptoms of Unruptured Intracranial Aneurysms. Stroke 2021;52(1):213–22.

83. Kang H, Tian DC, Yang X, et al. A Randomized Controlled Trial of Statins to Reduce Inflammation in Unruptured Cerebral Aneurysms. JACC Cardiovasc Imaging 2022;15(9):1668–70.

84. Edjlali M, Boulouis G, Derraz I, et al. Intracranial aneurysm wall enhancement decreases under anti-inflammatory treatment. Neurology 2018;91(17):804–5.

85. Zhang M, Peng F, Tong X, et al. Associations between haemodynamics and wall enhancement of intracranial aneurysm. Stroke Vasc Neurol 2021;6(3):467–75.

86. Hadad S, Mut F, Chung BJ, et al. Regional Aneurysm Wall Enhancement is Affected by Local Hemodynamics: A 7T MRI Study. AJNR Am J Neuroradiol 2021;42(3):464–70.

87. Raghuram A, Galloy A, Nino M, et al. Comprehensive morphomechanical analysis of brain aneurysms. Acta Neurochir 2023;165(2):461–70.

88. Larsen N, Fluh C, Saalfeld S, et al. Multimodal validation of focal enhancement in intracranial aneurysms as a surrogate marker for aneurysm

instability. Neuroradiology 2020. https://doi.org/10.1007/s00234-020-02498-6.

89. Khan MO, Toro Arana V, Rubbert C, et al. Association between aneurysm hemodynamics and wall enhancement on 3D vessel wall MRI. J Neurosurg 2020;10:1–11.

90. Calvin Gerald L, Alexandra L, Justin AM, et al. Performance of Radiomics derived morphological features for prediction of aneurysm rupture status. J Neurointerventional Surg 2021;13(8):755.

91. van Griethuysen JJM, Fedorov A, Parmar C, et al. Computational Radiomics System to Decode the Radiographic Phenotype. Cancer Res 2017;77(21):e104–7.

92. Veeturi S.S., Raghuram A., Miller J., et al., Radiomics Features in Contrast-Enhanced and Non-enhanced Magnetic Resonance Imaging Images Are Associated With High Intracranial Aneurysmal Risk. Stroke: Vascular and Interventional Neurology. 2023, 0(0):e000721. https://doi.org/10.1161/SVIN.122.000721.

93. Zhang Y, Ma C, Liang S, et al. Morphologic Feature Elongation Can Predict Occlusion Status Following Pipeline Embolization of Intracranial Aneurysms. World Neurosurg 2018;119:e934–40.

94. Liu Q, Jiang P, Jiang Y, et al. Prediction of Aneurysm Stability Using a Machine Learning Model Based on PyRadiomics-Derived Morphological Features. Stroke 2019;50(9):2314–21.

95. Ludwig CG, Lauric A, Malek JA, et al. Performance of Radiomics derived morphological features for prediction of aneurysm rupture status. J Neurointerv Surg 2021;13(8):755–61.

96. Chyatte D, Bruno G, Desai S, Todor DR. Inflammation and intracranial aneurysms. Neurosurgery 1999;45(5):1137–46.

97. Wang GX, Xia C, Liu J, et al. The Relationship of Arterial Wall Enhancement Ratio on MRI with the Degree of Inflammation in a Rabbit Aneurysm Model: A Pilot Study. Acad Radiol 2019;26(10):e292-e297.

Dual-Energy Computed Tomography in the Evaluation and Management of Subarachnoid Hemorrhage, Intracranial Hemorrhage, and Acute Ischemic Stroke

Joseph J. Gemmete, MD, FACR, FSIR, FCIRSE, FAHA*

KEYWORDS

- Dual energy computed tomography • Subarachnoid hemorrhage • Intracranial hemorrhage
- Acute ischemic stroke • Computed tomography

KEY POINTS

- Dual-energy computed tomography (DECT) is a valuable tool in the diagnosis and management of hemorrhage and ischemic stroke.
- DECT employs 2 distinct x-ray energy spectra to acquire images.
- The main advantage of DECT in the evaluation of subarachnoid hemorrhage (SAH) is its ability to differentiate between true SAH and mimics, such as contrast extravasation or venous congestion.
- One of the key advantages of DECT in intracranial hemorrhage is its ability to differentiate between hemorrhage and other hyperattenuating lesions, such as calcifications.
- In acute ischemic stroke, DECT can provide valuable information on the presence and extent of ischemia through the generation of iodine maps and perfusion maps.

INTRODUCTION

Cerebrovascular diseases, such as subarachnoid hemorrhage (SAH), intracranial hemorrhage (ICH), and acute ischemic stroke (AIS), are significant causes of morbidity and mortality worldwide. Rapid and accurate diagnosis is crucial to guide appropriate treatment and improve patient outcomes. While conventional computed tomography has been the mainstay of imaging in these patients, dual-energy CT (DECT) offers potential advantages in terms of sensitivity and specificity, as well as providing additional functional information.

PRINCIPLES OF DUAL-ENERGY COMPUTED TOMOGRAPHY

DECT is an advanced imaging modality that employs 2 distinct x-ray energy spectra to acquire images. This technology was first introduced by Hounsfield in 1973, but only recently has it become widely available in clinical practice.[1] DECT utilizes 2 x-ray sources and detectors that operate at different kilovoltage peak (kVp) settings, typically around 80 and 140 kVp, to capture images at high and low energy levels simultaneously.[2] Alternatively, rapid kVp switching can be utilized in

Departments of Radiology, Neurosurgery, Neurology, and Otolaryngology, Michigan Medicine, UH B1D 328, 1500 E Medical Center Drive, Ann Arbor, MI 48019, USA
* Corresponding author.
E-mail address: gemmete@med.umich.edu

Neuroimag Clin N Am 34 (2024) 241–249
https://doi.org/10.1016/j.nic.2023.12.001
1052-5149/24/© 2023 Elsevier Inc. All rights reserved.

neuroimaging.theclinics.com

single-source DECT systems to achieve a similar effect[3] (Fig. 1A–D).

The main advantage of DECT is its ability to generate material-specific data through material decomposition. This is achieved by exploiting the unique attenuation characteristics of different materials at varying x-ray energy levels. Based on these properties, DECT enables the differentiation and quantification of materials such as iodine, calcium, and blood products.[4]

DECT provides several postprocessing techniques to enhance image interpretation, including virtual non-contrast (VNC) images, monochromatic images, and material-specific maps. VNC images simulate traditional non-contrast CT images by removing the contribution of iodinated contrast, allowing for the evaluation of the native attenuation of tissues.[5] Monochromatic images can be generated at various keV levels, which can help optimize image quality, reduce beam-hardening artifacts,

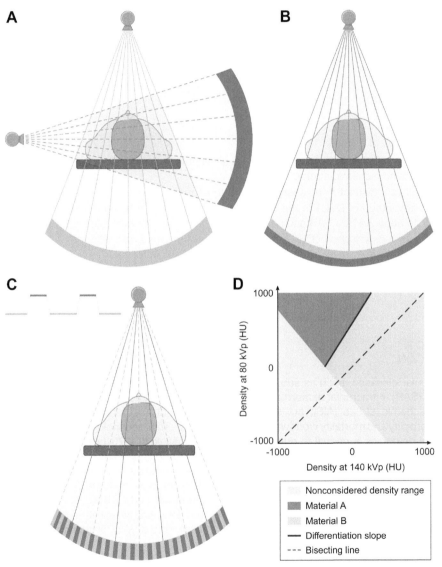

Fig. 1. (A) Sketch of dual-source CT system with two tubes and detectors mounted orthogonally in one gantry. (B) Sketch of layer detector system with one x-ray tube running at constant voltage. Dual-energy information is derived from two layers of detector with different sensitivity profiles. (C) Sketch of rapid kilovoltage-switching system containing only one tube and one detector. Voltage is switched rapidly between two levels. (D) Diagram of postprocessing algorithm – this algorithm is used to differentiate two materials from one another. Slope defines separation based on difference in densities of two materials in Hounsfield units. Two materials are color-coded in purple and light green.

and improve contrast-to-noise ratio (CNR).[6] Material-specific maps, such as iodine maps, can be generated to quantify the distribution of contrast material within tissues, providing additional functional information.[7]

DUAL-ENERGY COMPUTED TOMOGRAPHY IN SUBARACHNOID HEMORRHAGE

SAH is a life-threatening condition characterized by the extravasation of blood into the subarachnoid space. Accurate and timely diagnosis of SAH is crucial for appropriate management and improved patient outcomes. Conventional CT is the first-line imaging modality for detecting SAH; however, DECT has shown potential for improving diagnostic accuracy and providing additional information in this setting.[8]

One of the main advantages of DECT in the evaluation of SAH is its ability to differentiate between true SAH and mimics, such as contrast extravasation or venous congestion, which can appear similar on conventional CT (Fig. 2A, B). This is achieved through the generation of iodine maps and VNC images, which allow for the visualization of the native attenuation of tissues, thus improving diagnostic confidence and accuracy.[9,10]

DECT can also help in the evaluation of intracranial aneurysms, a common cause of SAH. By providing detailed information on the size, morphology, and relationship of aneurysms to surrounding structures, DECT can aid in surgical planning and endovascular treatment. DECT angiography has been shown to have a high sensitivity and specificity for detecting intracranial aneurysms and can be particularly

helpful in cases of SAH with negative initial digital subtraction angiography (DSA).[11–13]

Moreover, DECT can help identify the source of bleeding in patients with non-aneurysmal SAH, such as those caused by arteriovenous malformations (AVMs), dural arteriovenous fistulas (DAVFs), or other vascular pathologies, thus guiding appropriate management (Fig. 3A–D).[14]

DUAL-ENERGY COMPUTED TOMOGRAPHY IN INTRACRANIAL HEMORRHAGE

ICH is a severe cerebrovascular event that involves bleeding within the cranial cavity. Rapid and accurate diagnosis is essential for the appropriate management of ICH. Conventional CT has been the primary imaging modality for detecting ICH; however, DECT has demonstrated potential for improving diagnostic capabilities and providing valuable additional information in this setting (Fig. 4A–C).[15]

One of the key advantages of DECT in ICH is its ability to differentiate between hemorrhage and other hyperattenuating lesions, such as calcifications. This can be particularly useful in cases where it is difficult to differentiate between the 2 on conventional CT images (Fig. 5A, B).[16] DECT can also be utilized to identify active bleeding within the hematoma, which may be an important factor in determining the need for surgical intervention or conservative management.[17,18]

DECT can provide insights into the underlying etiology of ICH, such as vascular malformations or tumors. Material decomposition capabilities of DECT allow for better visualization of vascular

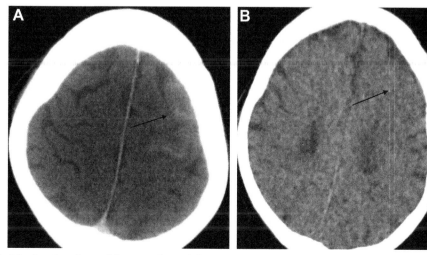

Fig. 2. CT of the head performed for neurological changes one hour after coiling of an ICA aneurysm. (*A*) Axial CT of the head shows an area of high attenuation in the left frontal region (*black arrow*). (*B*) Axial CT of the head iodine subtracted image shows no area of high attenuation (*black arrow*) consistent with contrast staining in the left frontal lobe NOT hemorrhage.

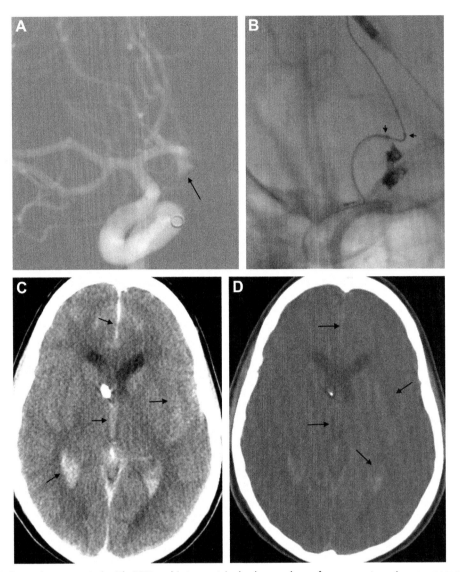

Fig. 3. Patient who presented with SAH and intraventricular hemorrhage from a rupture Acomm aneurysm. (*A*) RICA angiogram shows the boot shaped aneurysm involving the Acomm artery (*black arrow*). (*B*) Spot fluoroscopic image shows balloon across the neck of the aneurysm (*small black arrows*) with coils in the aneurysm and some outside the confines based on the initial angiogram. During coiling of the aneurysm there was an intraoperative rupture. (*C*) Axial CT of the head obtained immediately after coil embolization of the aneurysm shows diffuse high attenuation material in the ventricular system, interhemispheric fissure and sylvian fissure (*black arrows*). (*D*) Axial CT of the head iodine subtract image shows areas of decrease to absent high attenuation material in the ventricular system, interhemispheric fissure and sylvian fissure (*black arrows*) suggesting the material present of the initial regular CT of the head is contrast material not further hemorrhage.

structures and the detection of abnormal vascular connections, thus aiding in the diagnosis of AVMs or DAVFs.[19] In cases of suspected tumoral bleeding, DECT can help to differentiate between hemorrhage and tumor enhancement, guiding further management and treatment.[20]

Furthermore, DECT can be used to assess the extent of brain edema and mass effect associated with ICH, which may have prognostic implications

and help guide therapeutic decisions, such as decompressive craniectomy.[21]

DUAL-ENERGY COMPUTED TOMOGRAPHY IN ACUTE ISCHEMIC STROKE

AIS is a leading cause of morbidity and mortality worldwide. Rapid and accurate diagnosis is critical for the timely initiation of appropriate treatment,

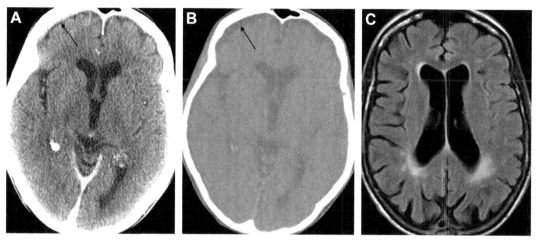

Fig. 4. CT of the head performed after a patient fall. (*A*) Axial CT of the head shows a crescent shaped area of high attenuation in the right frontal lobe (*black arrow*). The patient had a contrast enhanced CT of the abdomen and pelvic two hours prior to this exam for abdominal pain. (*B*) Axial CT of the head iodine subtract image (*black arrow*) shows no area of high attenuation. (*C*) Corresponding Axial FLAIR MRI image shows no acute subdural hematoma. The initial CT suggested a possible acute subdural hematoma which was subsequently shown not be present on the iodine subtract image and MRI.

such as thrombolytic therapy or endovascular intervention. Conventional CT and CT angiography have been the primary imaging modalities in the initial evaluation of AIS; however, DECT has demonstrated potential advantages in the diagnosis, management, and prognostication of patients with AIS (Fig. 6A, B).[22,23]

In AIS, DECT can provide valuable information on the presence and extent of ischemia through the generation of iodine maps and perfusion maps. These maps can help identify ischemic penumbra, which represents the salvageable brain tissue at risk of infarction if not reperfused in a timely manner.[24] This information can be crucial in selecting patients for reperfusion therapy and can help predict patient outcomes.[25]

DECT can also provide insights into the collateral circulation, which plays an essential role in maintaining blood flow to the ischemic penumbra. Studies have shown that the assessment of collateral circulation using DECT is highly correlated with the conventional DSA.[26] This information

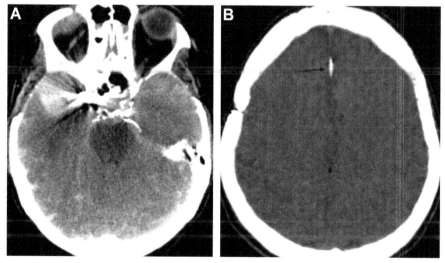

Fig. 5. CT of the head performed two hours after a myelogram for an acute severe headache. (*A*) Axial CT of the head shows diffuse high attenuation material predominantly in the subarachnoid space from the myelogram. (*B*) Axial CT of the head iodine subtract image at a different level shows high attenuation material in the interhemispheric fissure consistent with hemorrhage.

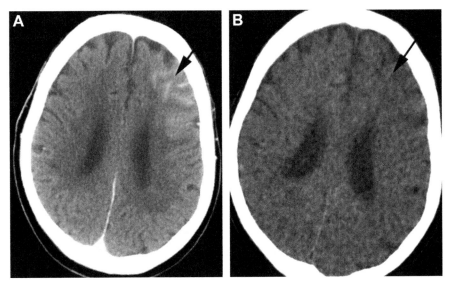

Fig. 6. CT of the head performed four hours after mechanical thrombectomy for a left middle cerebral artery occlusion. (*A*) Axial CT of the head shows an area of high attenuation in the left frontal region (*black arrow*). (*B*) Axial CT of the head iodine subtract images shows no area of high attenuation (*black arrow*) consistent with contrast staining in the area of tissue ischemia from breakdown of the blood brain barrier NOT hemorrhage.

can aid in the identification of patients who may benefit from endovascular treatment or other reperfusion strategies.[27]

Furthermore, DECT can help differentiate AIS from other stroke mimics, such as hemorrhagic transformation or tumor. This is particularly important in the acute setting, as the management of these conditions differs significantly from that of AIS.[28,29]

Lastly, DECT can be used to assess the degree of vascular calcification, which has been associated with an increased risk of complications during endovascular treatment, such as distal embolization or vessel perforation.[10] Furthermore, DECT may enable an improved visualization of ischemic brain tissue after mechanical thrombectomy in AIS.[30]

ADVANTAGES OF DUAL-ENERGY COMPUTED TOMOGRAPHY OVER CONVENTIONAL COMPUTED TOMOGRAPHY

DECT offers several advantages over conventional CT in various clinical scenarios, including neurovascular applications. Some of the main benefits of DECT include material decomposition, reduced beam-hardening artifacts, improved CNR, and the ability to generate VNC images.[4]

Material Decomposition

DECT leverages the unique attenuation characteristics of materials at different x-ray energy levels, enabling the differentiation and quantification of

various substances, such as iodine, calcium, and blood products.[2] This capability is valuable in distinguishing between different pathologies that may appear similar on conventional CT, such as differentiating ICH from contrast staining or calcifications.[8,31]

Reduced Beam-Hardening Artifacts

DECT allows for the generation of monochromatic images at various keV levels, which can help minimize beam-hardening artifacts that may obscure underlying pathology in conventional CT.[32] This advantage can be particularly useful in the evaluation of patients with intracranial hardware or calcifications.[33–35]

Improved Contrast-to-Noise Ratio

DECT can provide better CNR compared to conventional CT by optimizing the energy level at which images are generated. This results in improved image quality and enhanced visualization of subtle pathologies.[36,37]

Virtual Non-Contrast Images

DECT can generate VNC images by removing the contribution of iodinated contrast material. VNC images simulate traditional non-contrast CT images, allowing for the evaluation of the native attenuation of tissues.[38] This capability can be beneficial in differentiating between true pathology and contrast enhancement, as well as reducing radiation exposure by potentially eliminating the need for additional non-contrast CT scans in certain clinical situations.[39–41]

LIMITATIONS OF DUAL-ENERGY COMPUTED TOMOGRAPHY

Despite its numerous advantages, DECT also has several limitations that need to be considered when evaluating its role in neurovascular imaging.

Increased Radiation Dose

DECT can potentially lead to a higher radiation dose compared to conventional CT, especially when both low-energy and high-energy scans are acquired separately. However, recent advances in DECT technology, such as single-source DECT and advanced postprocessing algorithms, have helped mitigate this issue and optimize dose efficiency.[42,43]

Limited Availability

DECT scanners are not as widely available as conventional CT scanners, which may limit their accessibility for routine clinical use. Additionally, DECT technology often requires a higher initial investment compared to conventional CT systems.[44]

Image Noise and Artifacts

DECT images can be affected by increased image noise and artifacts, particularly at lower energy levels, which can impact image quality and diagnostic confidence. The use of advanced postprocessing techniques, such as noise reduction algorithms, can help address this issue.[45]

Complexity of Image Interpretation

DECT generates a large volume of data and multiple image sets, which can make image interpretation more complex and time-consuming compared to conventional CT. This may require additional training and expertise for radiologists to accurately interpret DECT images.[46]

Vendor-Specific Technology

DECT technology and postprocessing software are often vendor-specific, which can limit the ability to compare results between different scanner models and manufacturers. This also makes it challenging to establish standardized protocols and guidelines for DECT imaging.

SUMMARY

DECT has shown promise in the evaluation and management of cerebrovascular diseases, such as SAH, ICH, and AIS. By providing additional functional information and improving diagnostic accuracy, DECT can help guide appropriate treatment and improve patient outcomes. Further research is needed to explore its full potential and establish its role in the clinical setting.

CLINICS CARE POINTS

- DECT in the evaluation of SAH can differentiate between true SAH and mimics, such as contrast extravasation or venous congestion.
- DECT in ICH can differentiate between hemorrhage and other hyperattenuating lesions.
- DECT can provide information on the presence and extent of the cerebral ischemia.

DISCLOSURE

None.

REFERENCES

1. Hounsfield GN. Computerized transverse axial scanning (tomography). 1. Description of system. Br J Radiol 1973;46:1016–22.
2. Johnson TR. Dual-energy CT: general principles. AJR Am J Roentgenol 2012;199:S3–8.
3. Flohr TG, McCollough CH, Bruder H, et al. First performance evaluation of a dual-source CT (DSCT) system. Eur Radiol 2006;16:256–68.
4. McCollough CH, Leng S, Yu L, et al. Dual- and multi-energy CT: principles, technical approaches, and clinical applications. Radiology 2015;276:637–53.
5. Yu L, Christner JA, Leng S, et al. Virtual monochromatic imaging in dual-source dual-energy CT: radiation dose and image quality. Med Phys 2011;38:6371–9.
6. Kalender WA, Perman WH, Vetter JR, et al. Evaluation of a prototype dual-energy computed tomographic apparatus. I. Phantom studies. Med Phys 1986;13:334–9.
7. Graser A, Johnson TR, Hecht EM, et al. Dual-energy CT in patients suspected of having renal masses: can virtual nonenhanced images replace true nonenhanced images? Radiology 2009;252:433–40.
8. Phan CM, Yoo AJ, Hirsch JA, et al. Differentiation of hemorrhage from iodinated contrast in different intracranial compartments using dual-energy head CT. AJNR Am J Neuroradiol 2012;33:1088–94.
9. Boll DT, Patil NA, Paulson EK, et al. Renal stone assessment with dual-energy multidetector CT and advanced postprocessing techniques: improved

characterization of renal stone composition–pilot study. Radiology 2009;250:813–20.

10. Tijssen MP, Hofman PA, Stadler AA, et al. The role of dual energy CT in differentiating between brain haemorrhage and contrast medium after mechanical revascularisation in acute ischaemic stroke. Eur Radiol 2014;24:834–40.

11. Ni QQ, Tang CX, Zhao YE, et al. Single phase dual-energy CT angiography: one-stop-shop tool for evaluating aneurysmal subarachnoid hemorrhage. Sci Rep 2016;6:26704.

12. Mocanu I, Van Wettere M, Absil J, et al. Value of dual-energy CT angiography in patients with treated intracranial aneurysms. Neuroradiology 2018;60: 1287–95.

13. Stanton M, Sparti G. Use of dual-energy computed tomography post endovascular treatment of cerebral aneurysm. Surg Neurol Int 2021;12:225.

14. Guo Y, Ou SX, Qian M, et al. Dual-energy CT angiography for the diagnosis of intracranial dural arteriovenous fistula. Int J Clin Exp Med 2015;8:7802–8.

15. Dinkel J, Khalilzadeh O, Phan CM, et al. Technical limitations of dual-energy CT in neuroradiology: 30-month institutional experience and review of literature. J Neurointerventional Surg 2015;7:596–602.

16. Pomerantz SR, Kamalian S, Zhang D, et al. Virtual monochromatic reconstruction of dual-energy unenhanced head CT at 65-75 keV maximizes image quality compared with conventional polychromatic CT. Radiology 2013;266:318–25.

17. Peeters MTJ, Kort KJD, Houben R, et al. Dual-Energy CT Angiography Improves Accuracy of Spot Sign for Predicting Hematoma Expansion in Intracerebral Hemorrhage. J Stroke 2021;23:82–90.

18. Tan CO, Lam S, Kuppens D, et al. Spot and diffuse signs: quantitative markers of intracranial hematoma expansion at dual-energy CT. Radiology 2019;290: 179–86.

19. Potter CA, Sodickson AD. Dual-energy CT in emergency neuroimaging: added value and novel applications. Radiographics 2016;36:2186–98.

20. Choi Y, Shin NY, Jang J, et al. Dual-energy CT for differentiating acute intracranial hemorrhage from contrast staining or calcification: a meta-analysis. Neuroradiology 2020;62:1617–26.

21. Bodanapally UK, Shanmuganathan K, Gunjan YP, et al. Quantification of iodine leakage on dual-energy ct as a marker of blood-brain barrier permeability in traumatic hemorrhagic contusions: prediction of surgical intervention for intracranial pressure management. AJNR Am J Neuroradiol 2019;40:2059–65.

22. Naruto N, Itoh T, Noguchi K. Dual energy computed tomography for the head. Jpn J Radiol 2018;36: 69–80.

23. Itoh T, Noguchi K. Evaluation of the quantitative performance of non-enhanced dual-energy CT X-map in detecting acute ischemic brain stroke: A model observer study using computer simulation. Phys Med 2022;104:85–92.

24. Goyal M, Menon BK, van Zwam WH, et al. Endovascular thrombectomy after large-vessel ischaemic stroke: a meta-analysis of individual patient data from five randomised trials. Lancet 2016;387:1723–31.

25. van Ommen F, Dankbaar JW, Zhu G, et al. Virtual monochromatic dual-energy CT reconstructions improve detection of cerebral infarct in patients with suspicion of stroke. Neuroradiology 2021;63: 41–9.

26. Postma AA, Hofman PA, Stadler AA, et al. Dual-energy CT of the brain and intracranial vessels. AJR Am J Roentgenol 2012;199:S26–33.

27. Mohammed MF, Marais O, Min A, et al. Unenhanced dual-energy computed tomography: visualization of brain edema. Invest Radiol 2018;53:63–9.

28. Sananmuang T, Agarwal M, Maleki F, et al. Dual energy computed tomography in head and neck imaging: pushing the envelope. Neuroimaging Clin N Am 2020;30:311–23.

29. Kamalian S, Lev MH, Pomerantz SR. Dual-energy computed tomography angiography of the head and neck and related applications. Neuroimaging Clin N Am 2017;27:429–43.

30. Grkovski R, Acu L, Ahmadli U, et al. Dual-energy computed tomography in stroke imaging : value of a new image acquisition technique for ischemia detection after mechanical thrombectomy. Clin Neuroradiol 2023;33(3):747–54.

31. Bodanapally UK, Archer-Arroyo KL, Dreizin D, et al. Dual-energy computed tomography imaging of head: virtual high-energy monochromatic (190 keV) images are more reliable than standard 120 kV images for detecting traumatic intracranial hemorrhages. J Neurotrauma 2019;36:1375–81.

32. Kuchenbecker S, Faby S, Sawall S, et al. Dual energy CT: how well can pseudo-monochromatic imaging reduce metal artifacts? Med Phys 2015;42: 1023–36.

33. Gibney B, Redmond CE, Byrne D, et al. A Review of the Applications of Dual-Energy CT in Acute Neuroimaging. Can Assoc Radiol J 2020;71:253–65.

34. Mera Fernandez D, Santos Armentia E, Bustos Fiore A, et al. The utility of dual-energy CT for metal artifact reduction from intracranial clipping and coiling. Radiologia (Engl Ed) 2018;60:312–9.

35. Barreto I, Pepin E, Davis I, et al. Comparison of metal artifact reduction using single-energy CT and dual-energy CT with various metallic implants in cadavers. Eur J Radiol 2020;133:109357.

36. Shuman WP, Green DE, Busey JM, et al. Dual-energy liver CT: effect of monochromatic imaging on lesion detection, conspicuity, and contrast-to-noise ratio of hypervascular lesions on late arterial phase. AJR Am J Roentgenol 2014;203:601–6.

37. Lennartz S, Laukamp KR, Neuhaus V, et al. Dual-layer detector CT of the head: Initial experience in visualization of intracranial hemorrhage and hypodense brain lesions using virtual monoenergetic images. Eur J Radiol 2018;108:177–83.

38. Kessner R, Sommer J, Grosse Hokamp N, et al. Virtual versus true non-contrast images of the brain from spectral detector CT: comparison of attenuation values and image quality. Acta Radiol 2023;64:776–83.

39. Riederer I, Fingerle AA, Baum T, et al. Acute infarction after mechanical thrombectomy is better delineable in virtual non-contrast compared to conventional images using a dual-layer spectral CT. Sci Rep 2018;8:9329.

40. Nelles C, Laukamp KR, Grosse Hokamp N, et al. Virtual non-contrast reconstructions improve differentiation between vascular enhancement and calcifications in stereotactic planning CT scans of cystic intracranial tumors. Eur J Radiol 2022;157:110583.

41. Yun SY, Heo YJ, Jeong HW, et al. Dual-energy CT angiography-derived virtual non-contrast images for follow-up of patients with surgically clipped aneurysms: a retrospective study. Neuroradiology 2019;61:747–55.

42. Leng S, Yu L, Fletcher JG, et al. Maximizing iodine contrast-to-noise ratios in abdominal CT imaging through use of energy domain noise reduction and virtual monoenergetic dual-energy CT. Radiology 2015;276:562–70.

43. Patino M, Prochowski A, Agrawal MD, et al. Material separation using dual-energy CT: current and emerging applications. Radiographics 2016;36:1087–105.

44. Toshav A. Economics of dual-energy ct: workflow, costs, and benefits. Semin Ultrasound CT MR 2022;43:352–4.

45. Lee S, Choi YH, Cho YJ, et al. Noise reduction approach in pediatric abdominal CT combining deep learning and dual-energy technique. Eur Radiol 2021;31:2218–26.

46. Tamm EP, Le O, Liu X, et al. How to incorporate dual-energy imaging into a high volume abdominal imaging practice. Abdom Radiol (NY) 2017;42:688–701.

MR Vessel Wall Imaging for Atherosclerosis and Vasculitis

Mohamad M. Alzein, BS[a], Abhinav Patel, MD[a],
Ramez N. Abdalla, MD, PhD[a,b,c], Donald R. Cantrell, MD, PhD[a,b],
Ali Shaibani, MD[a,b,d], Sameer A. Ansari, MD, PhD[a,b,d,e,]*

KEYWORDS

• Vessel wall • Atherosclerosis • Vasculitis • Review

KEY POINTS

• Conventional imaging modalities, such as computed tomography angiography, MR angiography, transcranial Doppler ultrasonography, and digital subtraction angiography, are utilized in evaluating intraluminal or intravascular pathology of the intracranial vessels.
• We attempt to discuss the benefits of vessel wall imaging, specifically in the setting of intracranial atherosclerotic disease and vasculitis.
• In the setting of intracranial atherosclerotic disease, vessel wall imaging provides valuable information regarding plaque location as well as plaque characteristics that may predict clinical outcomes.
• Vessel wall imaging can provide information regarding extent, treatment response, and biopsy targets for vasculitis cases.

INTRODUCTION

Conventional imaging modalities, such as computed tomography (CT) angiography (CTA), MR angiography (MRA), transcranial Doppler ultrasonography, and digital subtraction angiography (DSA), are utilized in evaluating intraluminal or intravascular pathology of the intracranial vessels.[1] CTA and MRA are first-line imaging techniques to study the proximal intracranial arteries but are limited in sensitivity for distal small vessel pathology.[2,3] The historical gold standard for luminal evaluation has been DSA. Although DSA can accurately delineate stenoses in both large and small distal arteries (spatial resolution <0.4 mm), it carries an inherent risk of transient ischemic attack (TIA)/stroke due to invasive endovascular catheter techniques.[4]

Limitations of luminal imaging techniques can lead to inaccurate diagnosis, evaluation, and risk stratification, as many cerebrovascular pathologies contain an extrinsic vessel wall component. Analysis of the vessel wall is vital due to similar luminal findings of different cerebrovascular pathologies.[5] In addition, luminal evaluation may not accurately portray the extent of disease involvement. In the setting of vasculitis, concentric contrast enhancement was detected in segments with normal luminal findings on CTA and MRA.[6] Disease progression may only be noticeable on vessel wall analysis, as in the case of vessel remodeling in intracranial atherosclerotic disease (ICAD). Initially, atherosclerotic disease may build outward, leaving the lumen unaffected. Although the lumen is unaffected, studies have associated outward remodeling with the development of symptomatic plaques.[7-9] As such, luminal imaging may not provide sufficient information to accurately determine the risk of certain pathologies.

[a] Department of Radiology, Northwestern University, Feinberg School of Medicine; [b] Department of Radiology, Lurie Children's Hospital; [c] Department of Radiology, Ain Shams University, Faculty of Medicine; [d] Department of Neurological Surgery, Northwestern University, Feinberg School of Medicine; [e] Department of Neurology, Northwestern University, Feinberg School of Medicine
* Corresponding author. Northwestern University, Feinberg School of Medicine, 676 N. St. Clair Street, Suite 800 Chicago, IL 60611-2927.
E-mail address: s-ansari@northwestern.edu

Neuroimag Clin N Am 34 (2024) 251–260
https://doi.org/10.1016/j.nic.2024.02.001
1052-5149/24/© 2024 Elsevier Inc. All rights reserved.

Due to conventional imaging's inherent limitations for vessel wall evaluation, there is a need for additional techniques.[10] High-resolution vessel MR wall imaging (MR-VWI) can provide information on vessel wall characteristics. In this review, we attempt to discuss the benefits of vessel wall imaging (VWI), specifically in the setting of ICAD and vasculitis.

MR VESSEL WALL IMAGING PROTOCOL

Intracranial MR-VWI represents an evolution of the black-blood MR imaging technique, historically utilized to evaluate atherosclerosis in extracranial carotid arteries. MR-VWI hinges on several factors: blood flow and cerebrospinal fluid (CSF) suppression, spatial resolution, and sequence acquisition time. Achieving a high contrast-to-noise ratio (CNR) is imperative for VWI. This is facilitated by blood flow suppression in the vessel lumen, and CSF suppression outside the vessel wall, which creates a substantial signal disparity between the extraluminal and intraluminal regions adjacent to the vessel wall, rendering it conspicuous. Three-dimensional turbo spin echo (TSE) sequences leverage intravoxel dephasing to realize black-blood MR imaging. These sequences are typically employed on a 3-T magnet and allow a more accurate evaluation of relatively small intracranial blood vessels due to their superior signal-to-noise ratio (SNR) compared to 1.5-T magnets.

For optimal results, VWI requires a high CNR and SNR-derived spatial resolution. The wall thickness of the vessels in the Circle of Willis is 0.2 to 0.3 mm, and it reduces significantly more distally. This is smaller than the isometric voxels typically used in MR-VWI, which range between 0.4 and 0.7 mm. Despite this limitation, it is possible to accurately separate the MR imaging signal from the vessel wall by employing the aforementioned techniques to suppress signals originating from blood and CSF within the voxel, thereby delineating the structure. The acquisition time for a 3D TSE VWI sequence can be a limiting factor. A whole-brain coverage MR-VWI study employing isometric voxels could take well over 10 minutes to perform. Alternatively, a thinner slab sequence providing coverage limited to the Circle of Willis and its branches would be completed in as little as 5 to 7 minutes. Acquisition times can also be shortened with a volumetric 3D sequence and then reformatting the isotropic data to make it possible to be viewed in any two-dimensional plane needed to evaluate the blood vessel, an advantage in the tortuous intracranial vasculature. While a smaller voxel size would allow for a higher-resolution study, this would result in notably higher acquisition times or require a higher field (>3T) magnet, reducing its practicability in a clinical setting.

INTRACRANIAL ATHEROSCLEROTIC DISEASE
Definition and Pathophysiology

Estimates of the prevalence of intracranial atherosclerosis varies across different populations, with an autopsy study of patients with fatal strokes estimating ICAD to range up to 50% and accounting for 5% to 10% of ischemic stroke, though with a higher percentage in African Americans and reportedly up to 30% to 50% in Asians.[11–13] The formation of atherosclerotic plaques spans across several stages, beginning with the infiltration of lipoproteins into the vessel wall. Among its components are connective tissue extracellular matrix, cholesterol, phospholipids, inflammatory cells, smooth muscle cells, and thrombotic material. The variety of components leads to heterogeneity in plaque structure and disease progression.[14] Evaluation of plaque characteristics through VWI may provide insight into the risk of rupture and guide clinical decision-making.

MR Vessel Wall Imaging Findings

High-resolution MR-VWI of ICAD plaques usually demonstrates eccentric (crescent-like) thickening of the arterial wall.[15] On T2-weighted imaging, larger plaques may appear as focal hyperintense signal abnormality, with hypointense signal just peripherally adjacent to the vessel lumen, and possibly a band-like, juxtaluminal, hyperintense signal.[16,17] Analogous to carotid VWI, intracranial plaque imaging characteristics correlate with histologic findings. The periluminal T1 or T2 hypointense signal correlates with the lipid necrotic core while the juxtaluminal T2 hyperintense signal represents the fibrotic cap.[18,19] ICAD-related plaque enhancement on postcontrast T1 TSE imaging is typically diagnostic with irregular and eccentric enhancement but can be variable depending on multiple factors such as symptomatic versus asymptomatic status, time from symptomatic presentation, contrast bolus timing, imaging technique, and qualitative versus quantitative assessment[10] (Fig. 1).

Plaque Locations

ICAD plaque development can occur in different locations along the vessel wall and is at least partially dependent on the anatomy of intracranial vessels, which can have implications for the likelihood of symptomatic presentations and treatment. In the basilar artery, atherosclerotic plaques were reportedly most common on the ventral wall.[20] In

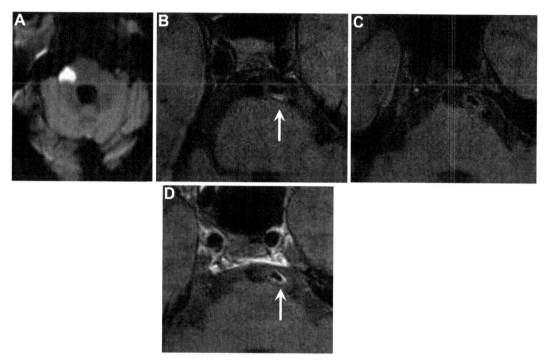

Fig. 1. Symptomatic atherosclerotic plaque of the basilar artery. (*A*) MR DWI identifies an acute perforator infarct in the right cerebellar-pontine angle. (*B*) Precontrast MR VWI demonstrates T1 hyperintense signal abnormality (*arrow*) along the posterior wall of the basilar artery, representing IPH. Precontrast (*C*) and postcontrast. (*D*) MR VWI demonstrates a separate region of eccentric vessel wall enhancement (*arrow*) of the basilar artery consistent with atherosclerotic plaque burden. MR DWI, magnetic resonance diffusion-weighted imaging.

the middle cerebral artery (MCA), one study found plaque involvement to be more likely in the ventral (44.8%) and inferior walls (31.7%), as compared to the superior (14.3%) and dorsal (9%) walls at the origin of lenticulostriate artery perforators.[21] In addition, plaque location was found to be different between symptomatic and asymptomatic plaques, with symptomatic MCA plaques more likely to be associated with superior wall locations.[21,22]

Plaque location may carry clinical significance in regard to prognosis and treatment outcomes such as with angioplasty/stenting. Angioplasty may result in a "snow plow" effect, in which plaque material can be pushed into small branching arteries, resulting in perforator occlusions and ischemic stroke complications. Determining the location of atherosclerotic plaques prior to angioplasty could potentially be utilized to determine angioplasty risk, although additional studies are required.[23]

Clinical Correlates

Atherosclerotic plaque heterogeneity likely leads to a spectrum of symptomatic presentations. A postmortem study reported causal atherothrombotic plaques causing between 30% and 75% stenosis of the vessel lumen. The variation in luminal stenosis within causal atherothrombotic plaques suggests the presence of contributing factors other than lumen stenosis.[11] Therefore, it is valuable to understand the clinical risks associated with ICAD imaging findings.

Intraplaque hemorrhage

Intraplaque hemorrhage (IPH) is thought to result from ruptured, fragile plaque neovasculature and appear as hyperintense signal abnormality within the plaque on T1-weighted VWI sequences.[24,25] In a study examining the prevalence of IPH in stenotic MCAs, it was reported in 10.1% of stenoses. Furthermore, symptomatic plaques—defined as an ischemic stroke in the distribution of the stenotic MCA—were more likely to present with IPH compared to asymptomatic plaques.[25] The association between IPH and symptomatic ICAD was corroborated by further studies.[24,26,27]

Lipid necrotic core

Progression of atherosclerotic plaques involves apoptosis of macrophage and smooth muscle cell-derived foam cells, which likely overwhelms the capabilities of local phagocytes. Lipid buildup results in the formation of a necrotic lipid core.[28] As previously stated, lipid necrotic cores appear as hypointense signal on both T1-weighted and T2-weighted MR-VWI sequences, due to the greater cholesterol than triglyceride plaque burden.[19] In a postmortem study assessing the morphologic features associated with stroke in atherosclerotic plaques, lipid area (>40%) was found to be an independent risk factor for MCA infarction.[29]

Compensatory remodeling

Blood vessels may respond to plaque burden through compensatory remodeling. Compensatory remodeling of arteries can be either outward (positive), which preserves luminal patency, or inward (negative), which constricts vessel lumen area and contributes to vessel stenosis.[30] Although positive remodeling preserves the luminal diameter, previous studies associated positive remodeling with an increased likelihood of symptomatic presentations and risk for downstream atheroemboli compared to constrictive negative remodeling.[7-9,31] For example, one study comparing symptomatic and asymptomatic ICAD plaques reported a greater likelihood of expansive remodeling in the symptomatic group—although the degree of stenosis was similar in both.[17]

Calcification

Calcification of atherosclerotic plaques can occur early in the disease process and accelerate as ICAD progresses. Calcification of atherosclerotic plaques is thought to occur through passive dystrophic calcification or active formation by smooth muscle cell-derived osteoblast-like cells.[32] It appears as hypointense signals on T1-weighted and T2-weighted MR-VWI sequences. The contribution of calcification to ICAD symptoms remains unclear due to a paucity of data in the intracranial literature. In one postmortem study, calcification was reported in up to 28% of plaques in the MCA—although the presence of calcification was not statistically different between plaques associated with infarcts and plaques that were not.[29] While not specific to MR-VWI, one study reported calcification on CT to be an independent risk factor for the presence of an ischemic stroke.[33]

Plaque enhancement

ICAD plaque enhancement may be utilized as a marker of plaque inflammation and neovascularization due to alterations in vascular permeability and subsequent gadolinium contrast uptake and visualization.[34] Symptomatic plaques have been shown to be associated with plaque enhancement in the territory of infarcts when compared with asymptomatic plaques.[34-36] As a result, plaque enhancement may reflect active plaques or plaque instability at risk for various ischemic stroke etiologies related to ICAD: in situ thrombosis with small vessel (perforator) occlusions, increasing plaque burden (stenosis) leading to hypoperfusion-related ischemia, and artery-to-artery emboli.

Along with predicting at risk plaques, enhancement in symptomatic plaques has been associated with specific infarction patterns and ischemic stroke mechanisms—specifically artery-to-artery embolic strokes. On the other hand, nonenhancing plaques had a heterogeneous distribution of stroke patterns consisting of thrombosis, small-vessel (perforator) occlusion, and arterial embolization.[37] Furthermore, another study reported similar findings and reported plaque enhancement as the strongest independent predictor of artery-to-artery embolic infarctions.[38]

Plaque enhancement may be utilized to track plaque evolution and treatment response, as it has been found to be greater in plaques associated with acute stroke (<4 weeks) and decreases in intensity over time.[39,40] Plaque enhancement's utility also extends to predicting recurrent stroke. A prospective, observational, longitudinal multicenter study aimed at investigating the predictive power of postcontrast atherosclerotic plaques of new strokes in symptomatic and asymptomatic patients reported a plaque enhancement ratio (defined as signal intensity of the plaque postcontrast/signal intensity of the corpus callosum) of greater than 1.77 was associated with new strokes in the future.[41] Similar results were confirmed in a second study, which demonstrated an increased enhancement ratio (defined as the slice of greatest enhancement and defined as the ratio between the normalized signal intensity of the plaque in CE-T1W and precontrast T1W images with reference to the nearby brain parenchyma) was associated with recurrent strokes in patients with symptomatic ICAD.[42]

Ferumoxytol

Inflammatory cells, namely macrophages, play a major role in the progression of atherosclerotic plaques. Ferumoxytol is a superparamagnetic oxide nanopeptide that is preferentially taken up by atherosclerotic plaques and cleared from the blood through macrophages.[43] As a result, it can be utilized as a marker for the presence of macrophages in atherosclerotic plaques and therefore possibly assess active inflammation.[44] Although its utility in intracranial atherosclerotic plaques has yet to be determined, one pilot study in the setting of cerebral aneurysms investigated the clinical relationship between early (<24 hours) and late (>72 hours) ferumoxytol uptake, reporting an increased likelihood of rupture in patients with early uptake.[45]

Pitfalls

Pathology mimics

Intracranial dissection Intracranial dissection presents with overlapping imaging findings, including eccentric wall thickening with enhancement.[10] Distinguishing characteristics would include T1 hyperintense wall elements on nonenhanced T1 fluid attenuated inversion recovery (FLAIR) sequences due to methemoglobin in the arterial wall and the presence of a false lumen[10] (Fig. 2). The double lumen may be more visible on T2-weighted and three dimensional-time of flight (3D-TOF) source images compared to T1-weighted images. In addition, intracranial dissections may present with an intimal flap, which can be seen as intraluminal linear hyperintensity on postcontrast T1-weighted and T2-weighted images versus hypointensity on 3D-TOF source.[46] Due to the overlap between imaging findings of intracranial atherosclerosis and dissection, the clinical presentation will be critical in aiding the diagnosis. Intracranial dissection should be considered in a previously healthy, younger individual presenting with neurologic deficits, possibly following minor head trauma, accompanied by headache or associated with connective tissue disease.[47]

Nonpathology mimics

Periarterial enhancement In addition to pathologic mimics, normal VWI findings may mimic pathology. Periarterial enhancement has been described and should be differentiated from pathologic findings. The location can provide data to distinguish from pathology, as it has been reported to be most common in the cavernous and petrous portion of the internal carotid artery, the intracranial V4 segments of the vertebral arteries, and the M1 segment of the MCA in a pediatric population. In addition, periarterial enhancement is more likely to be present symmetrically.[48]

Slow-flow artifacts In certain sequences that rely on the blood flow suppression of the intraluminal signal, slow-moving blood may appear as a mimic to wall thickening. This is due to the characteristic laminar blood flow, which demonstrates a relatively slower velocity of blood adjacent to the vessel wall compared to the center of the lumen and therefore inefficient suppression in this region. In addition, the slow flow from surrounding veins can contribute to the appearance of vessel wall thickening of nearby arteries.[49]

VASCULITIS

Definition and Pathophysiology

Vasculitis of the central nervous system (CNS) refers to the inflammation of the vasculature of the brain and spinal cord; it may also involve the meninges. Vasculitis may be restricted solely to the CNS, denoted as primary angiitis of the CNS, devoid of any systemic involvement. Conversely, it may emerge in the backdrop of a multitude of systemic inflammatory conditions, for example, infections or autoimmune processes.

MR Vessel Wall Imaging Findings

On postcontrast T1-weighted turbo spin echo imaging, vasculitis lesions typically manifest as a diffuse, circumferential vessel wall enhancement, possibly accompanied by wall thickening[10,50,51] (Fig. 3). Multiple arterial segments may be involved, which has been associated with likelihood of symptom relapse.[52] Luminal stenosis is common, and on rare occasions, eccentric enhancement commonly

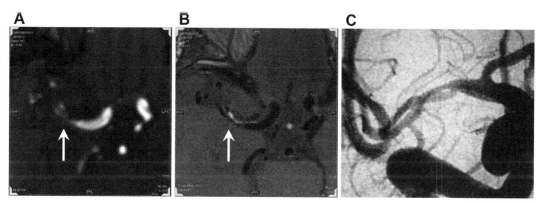

Fig. 2. Intracranial dissection of the M1 segment right MCA. (A) TOF MRA identifies a double lumen with central intimal flap (arrow). (B) Coregistration of postcontrast MR VWI T1 TSE sequence and (C) DSA imaging clearly delineates dual lumen pathology with intimal flap enhancement (arrow) or linear filling defect in the M1 segment, consistent with spiral intracranial dissection.

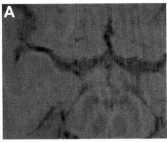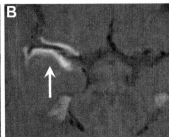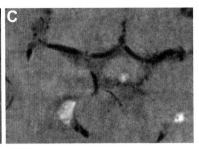

Fig. 3. Precontrast (*A*) and postcontrast (*B*) MR VWI demonstrates prominent, concentric vessel wall enhancement in the M1 segment of the right MCA (*arrow*), consistent with large-vessel cerebral vasculitis and confirmed with CSF analysis on lumbar puncture. (*C*) Six month follow-up postcontrast MR-VWI following after treatment demonstrates resolved concentric wall enhancement in the right MCA, consistent with corticosteroid response.

associated with atherosclerotic plaques may be perceived.

Clinical Applications

Diagnosis

In the setting of vasculitis, circumferential wall enhancement is thought to be due to inflammatory infiltrates in the endothelial lining.[53] The presence of vessel wall enhancement is relatively common, with one cerebral vasculitis study that analyzed 99 arterial segments and identified 92 with grade 2 enhancement as well as the remaining 7 with grade 1 enhancement.[52] The degree of enhancement may provide insight into prognosis, as lower enhancement grades have been associated with improved symptoms following treatment.[54]

Follow-up and treatment

VWI may be an invaluable tool in determining the risk of relapse as well as following response to treatment. MR-VWI can provide information into the extent of the disease, such as the location of involvement and the number of arterial segments, which has been associated with an increased risk of relapse.[52] In addition, it may be utilized as a tool to assess the improvement or resolution of disease on follow-up after treatment.[52,55]

Targeting biopsies

The gold standard for diagnosing CNS vasculitis is the histopathological biopsy of brain tissue, which typically reveals transmural inflammatory infiltrates. However, the invasive nature and relatively low sensitivity due to patchy involvement of the vessel wall underscore its inherent limitations.[56] Furthermore, the morbidity and mortality in these patients is substantial, necessitating prompt therapeutic interventions to mitigate adverse outcomes. Consequently, accurately diagnosing CNS vasculitis remains a formidable challenge.

VWI may provide additional support in the diagnosis of CNS vasculitis to guide biopsy site.[56,57] In a study by Zeiler and colleagues, MR-VWI was utilized to determine biopsy sites in 9 patients with clinical suspicion of CNS vasculitis. Of which, 8 biopsy sites were found to confirm inflammatory vasculitis for a definitive diagnosis.[56]

Pitfalls

Pathology mimics

Reversible cerebral vasoconstriction syndrome Differentiation between reversible cerebral vasoconstriction syndrome (RCVS) and vasculitis is necessary due to similar clinical presentations but different treatments. While vasculitis is treated with steroids and immunosuppressive therapies, RCVS is treated with conservative medical management with calcium channel blockers. RCVS is likely due to arterial tone dysregulation, and the limited histologic data suggest a lack of an inflammatory component.[58] Cerebral vasculitis and RCVS are similar in that they both present with concentric wall thickening on MR-VWI. However, as opposed to the diffuse, intense enhancement pattern seen with vasculitis, RCVS usually presents with mild-to-no enhancement on MR-VWI.[59,60]

Moyamoya disease Moyamoya disease (MMD) is an idiopathic, cerebrovascular disease that presents as a progressive steno-occlusive vasculopathy of the distal internal carotid artery (ICA) and proximal Circle of Willis segments.[61,62] Similarly to cerebral vasculitis, MMD usually presents with a concentric disease pattern[61,63] (Fig. 4). Although both vasculitis and MMD contain a concentric vessel wall thickening pattern, the location of the disease is mainly proximal at the distal ICA and its branches, and more likely bilateral in MMD. In addition, MMD is associated with the development of hypertrophied lenticulostriate and perforator collaterals at the base of the brain that are classically described as a "puff of smoke" pattern on DSA.[61–63] The degree of vessel wall enhancement in MMD likely differs from cerebral vasculitis, with

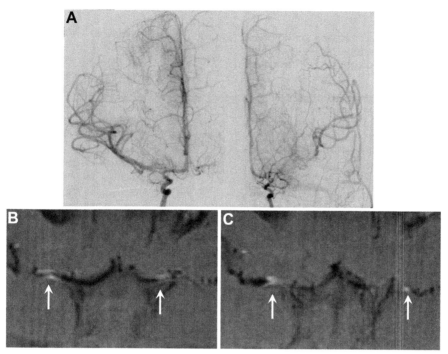

Fig. 4. (A) AP DSA images of bilateral carotid injections demonstrate severe narrowing in the bilateral supraclinoid internal carotid arteries and M1 middle cerebral arteries resulting in left M1 segment occlusion and compensating lenticulostriate collaterals, consistent with steno-occlusive vasculopathy/MMD. Precontrast (B) and postcontrast (C) MR VWI demonstrating confirms moderate-to-severe stenoses in these segments with circumferential enhancement in the bilateral M1 segments (arrows) suggesting inflammatory pathology in early MMD, as well as intraluminal enhancement of the left M1 segment, compatible with complete occlusion. AP, anteroposterior.

studies reporting minimal or absent enhancement of vessels, though it is unclear if there may be an inflammatory component to MMD in the early disease state.[10,64] However, absence of enhancement should be cautiously interpreted on imaging, as one study reported significantly greater enhancement in the ICAs of patients with MMD regardless of the presence of symptoms.

Nonpathology mimic

Circumferential segmental vessel-wall enhancement As the name suggests, circumferential segmental vessel-wall enhancement (CSWE) can be a mimic for vasculitis, presenting with concentric enhancement of the vessel wall. The phenomenon currently is thought to be due to the presence of the vasa vasorum or early atherosclerosis. Data describing its prevalence are limited. Although one study reported the presence of CSWE in the posterior circulation in 11 out of 12 patients and 5 out of 12 patients in the anterior circulation. With the posterior circulation further divided, V4 vertebral arteries (67%) and basilar segments (33%) had the highest prevalence of CSWE.[65]

SUMMARY

High-resolution MR VWI is an evolving field, providing information on cerebrovascular pathologies that extend beyond luminal characteristics. Additional information provided by MR-VWI can aid in diagnosis of similar pathologies, predict progression of disease, and monitor treatment response. While MR VWI can provide robust data on vessel wall characteristics, further prospective, multicenter studies are required to improve diagnostic accuracy and application.

CLINICS CARE POINTS

- Luminal or angiographic imaging modalities are relatively non-specific in diagnosing specific cerebrovascular pathologies, and therefore, MR vessel wall imaging (VWI) can provide important information to improve diagnostic accuracy, most commonly intracranial atherosclerotic disease (ICAD) and vasculitis.

- Various normal anatomic and pathological mimics must be considered when attempting to using MR VWI to diagnose cerebrovascular pathology.
- The pattern and degree of contrast enhancement on MR VWI may not only assist in the diagnosis of symptomatic ICAD and vasculitis, but may also predict treatment response.

DISCLOSURE

The authors have no disclosures with respect to conflicts of interest to report.

ACKNOWLEDGMENTS

National Institute of Neurological Disorders and Stroke (1R01NS114632) National Heart, Lung and Blood Institute (1R01HL149787).

REFERENCES

1. Ryu C-W, Jahng G-H, Kim E-J, et al. High Resolution Wall and Lumen MRI of the Middle Cerebral Arteries at 3 Tesla. Cerebrovasc Dis 2009;27(5):433–42.
2. Nguyen-Huynh MN, Wintermark, English, et al. How Accurate Is CT Angiography in Evaluating Intracranial Atherosclerotic Disease? Stroke 2008;39(4):1184–8.
3. Bash S, Villablanca JP, Jahan R, et al. Intracranial Vascular Stenosis and Occlusive Disease: Evaluation with CT Angiography, MR Angiography, and Digital Subtraction Angiography. AJNR Am J Neuroradiol 2005;26(5):1012–21.
4. Cloft HJ, Joseph GJ, Dion JE. Risk of Cerebral Angiography in Patients With Subarachnoid Hemorrhage, Cerebral Aneurysm, and Arteriovenous Malformation: A Meta-Analysis. Stroke 1999;30(2):317–20.
5. Li M, Xu, Song, et al. Atherosclerosis of middle cerebral artery: Evaluation with high-resolution MR imaging at 3T. Atherosclerosis 2009;204:447–52.
6. Destrebecq V, Sadeghi, Lubicz, et al. Intracranial Vessel Wall MRI in Cryptogenic Stroke and Intracranial Vasculitis. J Stroke Cerebrovasc Dis 2020;29:104684.
7. Qiao Y, Anwar, Intrapiromkul, et al. Patterns and Implications of Intracranial Arterial Remodeling in Stroke Patients. Stroke 2016;47:434–40.
8. Zhang D-F, Chen, Chen, et al. A High-Resolution MRI Study of Relationship between Remodeling Patterns and Ischemic Stroke in Patients with Atherosclerotic Middle Cerebral Artery Stenosis. Front Aging Neurosci 2017;9:140.
9. Chung GH, Kwak HS, Hwang SB, et al. High resolution MR imaging in patients with symptomatic middle cerebral artery stenosis. Eur J Radiol 2012;81:4069–74.
10. Swartz RH, Bhuta, Farb, et al. Intracranial arterial wall imaging using high-resolution 3-tesla contrast-enhanced MRI. Neurology 2009;72:627–34.
11. Mazighi M, Labreuche, Gongora-Rivera, et al. Autopsy Prevalence of Intracranial Atherosclerosis in Patients With Fatal Stroke. Stroke 2008;39(4):1142–7.
12. Suri MFK, Johnston SC. Epidemiology of Intracranial Stenosis. J Neuroimaging 2009;19 Suppl 1:11S–116S.
13. White H, Boden-Albala, Wang, et al. Ischemic Stroke Subtype Incidence Among Whites, Blacks, and Hispanics: The Northern Manhattan Study. Circulation 2005;111:1327–31.
14. Fuster V, Fayad PR, Moreno ZA, et al. Atherothrombosis and high-risk plaque: Part II: approaches by noninvasive computed tomographic/magnetic resonance imaging. J Am Coll Cardiol 2005;46:1209–18.
15. Klein IF, Lavallée PC, Touboul PJ, et al. In vivo middle cerebral artery plaque imaging by high-resolution MRI. Neurology 2006;67:327–9.
16. Klein IF, Lavallée PC, Schouman-Claeys E, et al. High-resolution MRI identifies basilar artery plaques in paramedian pontine infarct. Neurology 2005;64:551–2.
17. Xu W-H, Li, Gao, et al. In In vivo high-resolution MR imaging of symptomatic and asymptomatic middle cerebral artery atherosclerotic stenosis. Atherosclerosis 2010;212:507–11.
18. Majidi S, Sein, Watanabe, et al. Intracranial-Derived Atherosclerosis Assessment: An In Vitro Comparison between Virtual Histology by Intravascular Ultrasonography, 7T MRI, and Histopathologic Findings. AJNR Am J Neuroradiol 2013;34:2259–64.
19. van der Kolk AG, Zwanenburg, Denswil, et al. Imaging the Intracranial Atherosclerotic Vessel Wall Using 7T MRI: Initial Comparison with Histopathology. AJNR Am J Neuroradiol 2015;36(4):694–701.
20. Huang B, Yang, Liu, et al. Basilar artery atherosclerotic plaques distribution in symptomatic patients: A 3.0T high-resolution MRI study. Eur J Radiol 2013;82:e199, 203.
21. Xu W-H, Li, Gao, et al. Plaque Distribution of Stenotic Middle Cerebral Artery and Its Clinical Relevance. Stroke 2011;42(10):2957–9.
22. Zhu XJ, Du, Lou, et al. Morphologic Characteristics of Atherosclerotic Middle Cerebral Arteries on 3T High-Resolution MRI. AJNR Am J Neuroradiol 2013;34(9):1717–22.
23. Jiang W-J, Yu, Ma, et al. High resolution MRI guided endovascular intervention of basilar artery disease. J Neurointerv Surg 2011;3:375–8.
24. Zhu C, Tian, Degnan, et al. Clinical Significance of Intraplaque Hemorrhage in Low- and High-Grade Basilar Artery Stenosis on High-Resolution MRI. AJNR Am J Neuroradiol 2018;39:1286–92.

25. Xu W-H, Li, Gao, et al. Middle cerebral artery intraplaque hemorrhage: Prevalence and Clinical Relevance. Ann Neurol 2012;71:195–8.

26. Yu JH, Kwak, Chung, et al. Association of Intraplaque Hemorrhage and Acute Infarction in Patients With Basilar Artery Plaque. Stroke 2015;46:2768–72.

27. Yang W-Q, Huang, Liu, et al. Reproducibility of high-resolution MRI for the middle cerebral artery plaque at 3T. Eur J Radiol 2014;83:e49–55.

28. Buckley ML, Ramji DP. The influence of dysfunctional signaling and lipid homeostasis in mediating the inflammatory responses during atherosclerosis. Biochim Biophys Acta 2015;1852:1498–510.

29. Chen XY, Wong KS, Lam WWM, et al. Middle Cerebral Artery Atherosclerosis: Histological Comparison between Plaques Associated with and Not Associated with Infarct in a Postmortem Study. Cerebrovasc Dis 2008;25(1–2):74–80.

30. Glagov S, Weisenberg E, Zarins CK, et al. Compensatory Enlargement of Human Atherosclerotic Coronary Arteries. N Engl J Med 1987;316:1371–5.

31. Shi M-C, Wang, Zhou, et al. Compensatory remodeling in symptomatic middle cerebral artery atherosclerotic stenosis: a high-resolution MRI and microemboli monitoring study. Neurol Res 2012;34:153–8.

32. Doherty TM, Asotra, Fitzpatrick, et al. Calcification in atherosclerosis: Bone biology and chronic inflammation at the arterial crossroads. Proc Natl Acad Sci U S A 2003;100:11201–6.

33. Chen X, Lam WWM, Ng HK, et al. Intracranial Artery Calcification: A Newly Identified Risk Factor of Ischemic Stroke. J Neuroimaging 2007;17(4):300–3.

34. Vakil P, Vranic, Hurley, et al. T1 Gadolinium Enhancement of Intracranial Atherosclerotic Plaques Associated with Symptomatic Ischemic Presentations. AJNR Am J Neuroradiol 2013;34(12):2252–8.

35. Vergouwen MDI, Silver FL, Mandell DM, et al. Eccentric Narrowing and Enhancement of Symptomatic Middle Cerebral Artery Stenoses in Patients With Recent Ischemic Stroke. Arch Neurol 2011;68:338–42.

36. Qiao Y, Zeiler, Mirbagheri, et al. Intracranial Plaque Enhancement in Patients with Cerebrovascular Events on High-Spatial-Resolution MR Images. Radiology 2014;271(2):534–42.

37. Kim J-M, Jung, Sohn, et al. Middle Cerebral Artery Plaque and Prediction of the Infarction Pattern. Arch Neurol 2012;69(11):1470–5.

38. Wu F, Song, Ma, et al. Hyperintense Plaque on Intracranial Vessel Wall Magnetic Resonance Imaging as a Predictor of Artery-to-Artery Embolic Infarction. Stroke 2018;49:905–11.

39. Skarpathiotakis M, Mandell DM, Swartz RH, et al. Intracranial Atherosclerotic Plaque Enhancement in Patients with Ischemic Stroke. AJNR Am J Neuroradiol 2013;34:299–304.

40. Yang W-J, Abrigo, Soo, et al. Regression of Plaque Enhancement Within Symptomatic Middle Cerebral Artery Atherosclerosis: A High-Resolution MRI Study. Front Neurol 2020;11:755.

41. Gómez-Vicente B, Hernández-Pérez M, Marínez-Velasco E, et al. Intracranial atherosclerotic plaque enhancement and long-term risk of future strokes: A prospective, longitudinal study. J Neuroimaging 2023;33:289–301.

42. Yang D, Liu, Yao, et al. The MRI enhancement ratio and plaque steepness may be more accurate for predicting recurrent ischemic cerebrovascular events in patients with intracranial atherosclerosis. Eur Radiol 2022;32(10):7004–13.

43. Smits LP, Tiessens, Zheng, et al. Evaluation of ultrasmall superparamagnetic iron-oxide (USPIO) enhanced MRI with ferumoxytol to quantify arterial wall inflammation. Atherosclerosis 2017;263:211–8.

44. Trivedi RA, U-King-Im, Graves, et al. In In vivo detection of macrophages in human carotid atheroma: temporal dependence of ultrasmall superparamagnetic particles of iron oxide-enhanced MRI. Stroke 2004;35(7):1631–5.

45. Hasan D, Chalouhi, Jabbour, et al. Early Change in Ferumoxytol-Enhanced Magnetic Resonance Imaging Signal Suggests Unstable Human Cerebral Aneurysm: A Pilot Study. Stroke 2012;43(12):3258–65.

46. Wang Y, Lou, Li, et al. Imaging investigation of intracranial arterial dissecting aneurysms by using 3 T high-resolution MRI and DSA: from the interventional neuroradiologists' view. Acta Neurochir 2014;156:515–25.

47. Gao PH, Yang, Wang, et al. Symptomatic unruptured isolated middle cerebral artery dissection: clinical and magnetic resonance imaging features. Clin Neuroradiol 2016;26:81–91.

48. Mineyko A, Kirton A, Ng D, et al. Normal intracranial periarterial enhancement on pediatric brain MR imaging. Neuroradiology 2013;55:1161–9.

49. Lindenholz A, van der Kolk AG, Zwanenburg JJM, et al. The Use and Pitfalls of Intracranial Vessel Wall Imaging: How We Do It. Radiology 2018;286:12–28.

50. Obusez EC, Hui, Hajj-Ali, et al. High-Resolution MRI Vessel Wall Imaging: Spatial and Temporal Patterns of Reversible Cerebral Vasoconstriction Syndrome and Central Nervous System Vasculitis. AJNR Am J Neuroradiol 2014;35(8):1527–32.

51. Fan TH, Khoury, Cho, et al. Cerebrovascular complications and vasculopathy in patients with herpes simplex virus central nervous system infection. J Neurol Sci 2020;419:117200.

52. Yang X, Sun J, Jia M-Y, et al. The value of high-resolution MRI in the diagnosis, efficacy of treatment, and prognosis of central nervous system vasculitis. fn 2021;59(4):372–7.

53. Song JW, Shou, Obusez, et al. Spatial Distribution of Intracranial Vessel Wall Enhancement in Hypertension and Primary Angiitis of the CNS. Sci Rep 2019;9:19270.

54. Kang H, Bai, Zhang, et al. Predictors of improvement for patients with CNS vasculitis stenoses: A high-resolution vessel wall MRI follow-up study. Eur J Radiol 2023;158:110619.

55. Tsivgoulis G, Papadimitropoulos, Lachanis, et al. High-resolution Intracranial Vessel Wall Imaging in Monitoring Treatment Response in Primary CNS Angiitis. Neurol 2018;23:188–90.

56. Zeiler SR, Qiao Y, Pardo CA, et al. Vessel Wall MRI for Targeting Biopsies of Intracranial Vasculitis. AJNR Am J Neuroradiol 2018;39:2034–6.

57. Bley TA, Wieben, Uhl, et al. High-Resolution MRI in Giant Cell Arteritis: Imaging of the Wall of the Superficial Temporal Artery. AJR Am J Roentgenol 2005; 184(1):283–7.

58. Serdaru M, Chiras J, Cujas M, et al. Isolated benign cerebral vasculitis or migrainous vasospasm? J Neurol Neurosurg Psychiatry 1984;47:73–6.

59. Mandell DM, Matouk, Farb, et al. Vessel Wall MRI to Differentiate Between Reversible Cerebral Vasoconstriction Syndrome and Central Nervous System Vasculitis: Preliminary Results. Stroke 2012;43(3): 860–2.

60. Mossa-Basha M, Hwang, De Havenon, et al. Multicontrast High-Resolution Vessel Wall Magnetic Resonance Imaging and Its Value in Differentiating Intracranial Vasculopathic Processes. Stroke 2015; 46(6):1567–73.

61. Yuan M, Liu, Wang, et al. High-resolution MR imaging of the arterial wall in moyamoya disease. Neurosci Lett 2015;584:77–82.

62. Takagi Y, Kikuta K, Nozaki K, et al. Histological Features of Middle Cerebral Arteries From Patients Treated for Moyamoya Disease. Neurol Med -Chir 2007;47:1–4.

63. Ryoo S, Cha, Kim, et al. High-Resolution Magnetic Resonance Wall Imaging Findings of Moyamoya Disease. Stroke 2014;45(8):2457–60.

64. Aoki S, Hayashi, Abe, et al. Radiation-induced arteritis: thickened wall with prominent enhancement on cranial MR images report of five cases and comparison with 18 cases of Moyamoya disease. Radiology 2002;223(3):683–8.

65. Gaddam DS, Crews, Chryssikos, et al. Circumferential segmental vessel-wall enhancement on black blood MRI in patients referred for the evaluation of vasculopathy. Clin Imaging 2021;80:67–71.

Advances in Intraoperative Imaging for Vascular Neurosurgery

Chanju Fritch, MD, Ephraim Church, MD, David Andrew Wilkinson, MD, MS*

KEYWORDS

- Intraoperative imaging • Cerebral angiogram • Indocyanine green angiography
- Relative fluorescence measurement (FLOW 800)

KEY POINTS

- Digital subtraction angiography remains both a common modality and a gold standard modality for many open cerebrovascular surgeries.
- The addition of the hybrid operating room, or one with built-in angiographic capability, is a promising way to integrate real-time imaging into the procedural workflow.
- Indocyanine green angiography is useful in examination of a specific surgical field and helps in the assessment of flow within the visualized structures. It is limited when visibility is limited.
- Relative fluorescence measurement measures the time involved and the maximal peak of fluorescent signal within regions of interest. It is often used in arteriovenous malformation surgery, where flow dynamics can change significantly within the lesion during the course of the surgery.

 Video content accompanies this article at http://www.neuroimaging.theclinics.com.

INTRODUCTION

Identification, preservation, and manipulation of cerebrovascular architecture are key to safe vascular neurosurgery. Intraoperative imaging of neurosurgical disease represents an important adjunct to aid in surgical decision-making within this context. There are many modalities available, largely depending on the pathology receiving surgery. Intraoperative neurovascular imaging has its greatest impact in decision-making in the contexts of aneurysm surgery,[1] arteriovenous malformation (AVM) and arteriovenous fistula (AVF) surgery,[2] and cerebral bypass surgery.[3] In the following sections, the notable techniques utilized by neurosurgeons are reviewed.

TECHNIQUES
Intraoperative Digital Subtraction Angiography

Intraoperative digital subtraction angiography (DSA) was the original, remains one of the most familiar tools of the vascular neurosurgeon, and is the gold standard in characterization of aneurysms and AVM/AVFs.

When considering the use of intraoperative DSA, a radiolucent table and head-holder are necessary to allow optimal visualization.[4] Further instrumentation is often exchanged for radiolucent alternatives (eg, Hook and rubber band retraction in lieu of Greenberg retraction). Tradiionally, transfemoral access has been used,

Department of Neurosurgery, Penn State Milton S. Hershey Medical Center, 500 University Drive, Hershey, PA 17033, USA
* Corresponding author.
E-mail address: dwilkinson@pennstatehealth.psu.edu

Neuroimag Clin N Am 34 (2024) 261–270
https://doi.org/10.1016/j.nic.2024.01.005

though transradial access has become another popular option.

When the surgeon is ready for DSA (most often after aneurysm clipping or AVM resection), the angiographer (oftentimes also the primary surgeon) manipulates a diagnostic catheter into the relevant carotid or vertebral artery under fluoroscopic guidance, taking care that navigation may be more challenging due to atypical positioning. At key points of surgery, the surgeon will clear the operative field of unnecessary radiopaque instruments and the fluoroscope is introduced for performing the angiogram. In a traditional operating room, a typical C-arm with video fluoroscopy can be utilized for angiography. More recently, hybrid-ORs,[5] or an operating room with integrated wall/floor mounted fluoroscopy units, have found favor and utilization by neurosurgeons.

A "hybrid-OR" is one equipped with both a traditional surgical table and imaging equipment integrated into the walls, ceiling, and/or floor; this was first described in 1997 within the context of coronary artery bypass graft surgery and cardiac angiogram.[6] Since its arrival, the hybrid-OR has gained traction in nearly all surgical subspecialties, including neurosurgery. The benefits of a hybrid-OR are attractive; when correctly utilized, the hybrid-OR allows a surgeon to achieve a streamlined workflow to include real-time images in the patient's operative positioning. A recent meta-analysis found that neurosurgical hybrid ORs are used predominantly in the fields of cerebrovascular neurosurgery (including endovascular surgery) and in spine.[7] The most cited advantage of the hybrid-OR was the ability to assess an outcome during a critical surgical step and examples included safe clip placement, aneurysm obliteration, AVM resection, fistulae removal, and screw placement. The second most cited advantage was the ability to perform both endovascular and open portions of surgery at the same time without time-consuming patient transport and staffing accommodation. A subtle corollary of this feature was noted by the authors in the surgical team's ability to rapidly detect complications and improve patient safety as a result. Other advantages noted included improved accuracy of the procedure and general versatility of the room. Limitations noted included limited patient positioning (due to commitment to the room's nontraditional operating table), limitation in patient size because of the gantry size of the C-arm, radiation exposure with its associated monitoring and safety needs, the cumbersome nature of the imaging equipment, sterility, and the necessity of a larger space in general.

In cases where the patient is positioned supine, the femoral artery can be accessed in the traditional manner. Both preincision and postincision sheath placements are options for the surgical team. For cases requiring prone, three-fourths prone, or lateral positioning, access can be more difficult. One described solution is utilization of an extended femoral sheath that offers the angiographer an entry point separate from the patient's otherwise difficult to access groin.[8] In these cases, the extended sheath was placed while the patient was supine, the femoral site carefully dressed, the sheath itself secured, and then the patient repositioned. Before incision, the extended sheath's entrance is usually found immediately lateral to the patient's thigh.[9] It should be noted that angiogram was planned as a portion of the procedure a priori in these cases. Another described solution involved arterial access via the popliteal artery.[10] This access site had the advantage of being accessible even when an intraoperative angiogram was not planned presurgery, and the authors noted its utility in performing a spinal angiogram in the prone position. Another set of authors found a solution by utilizing the upper extremity as the site of arterial vascular access[11,12] (further discussion of transradial arterial access is included in the following section).

Within the context of open aneurysm surgery, that is, clipping of an aneurysm, preoperative DSA is used to identify critical perforators, adjacent normal vasculature, and aneurysm architecture. While this can be done before the day of surgery, some operators will perform their preoperative angiogram on the same day of the procedure with the patient in their intended positioning.[13] After placement of a clip, angiography is used to confirm patency of healthy vasculature and exclusion of the aneurysm from flow.[14] In this manner, angiography allows the neurosurgeon to identify residual aneurysm and decide whether to reposition the clip. Prior case series have cited rates between 8%[15] and 12%[16] for intraop DSA changing the course of surgery.

Within the context of AVM surgery, intraop DSA is typically used to confirm complete resection of the AVM nidus, and it can guide the neurosurgeon to re-engage the surgical bed to identify and resect residual malformation[17] (Fig. 1A and B). However, a later follow up DSA can sometimes reveal residual AVM when an operative DSA demonstrated no such residual; previously published case series cite an 8%[18] and 9%[2] rate of this occurring. Postsurgery angiography done in a delayed fashion demonstrated that the operative angiogram was falsely negative (ie, there was AVM

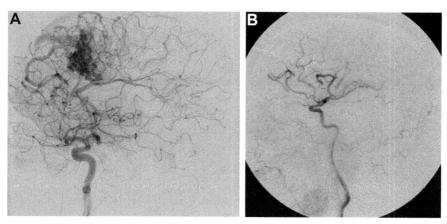

Fig. 1. (A) Preoperative DSA (lateral, arterial phase, left carotid injection) of a left frontal AVM. (B) Postresection intraoperative angiogram for the same lesion showing no residual AVM and patency of adjacent vessels.

left behind despite the encouraging imaging) in roughly 10% of cases,[2,18] although these were small studies. These data emphasize that a compromise is often made, favoring immediate intraoperative images with slightly lower quality compared with higher quality postoperative images in the full angiography suite; the use of true hybrid-ORs may negate some of this difference in image quality. Cerebral bypass surgery can also utilize intraoperative angiography to confirm patency of the bypass graft.[19] Other strategies (namely, ICG fluoroscopy) have gained popularity for this intervention as well.

While the transfemoral access site has been the historically cannulated vessel for angiography, some institutions are favoring radial (or even ulnar) access for their associated patient safety and satisfaction outcomes. Within the single-center case series cited, contrast and radiation doses were not significantly different between forearm and groin access sites.[20] Additionally, wrist access also facilitated angiography for prone or three-fourths turn positioned patients; one case series demonstrated feasibility of this combination in treatment of aneurysm, fistula, and malformation.[21] This is especially relevant in the treatment of spinal, occipital, or suboccipital pathologies. Another case series featured radial access for thoracic intraoperative spinal angiography without complication.[11]

Indocyanine Green Angiography

While DSA has been the traditional gold standard, more recently DSA has found competition in video indocyanine green (ICG) angiography because of ICG's ease of use and ability to forego vascular access/diagnostic catheter placement.[3] ICG originally found its home in medicine in the examination of retinal blood flow within ophthalmology; ICG is a tricarbocyanine dye that absorbs and reflects in the near infrared electromagnetic spectrum.[22,23] It undergoes an efficient first pass process at the liver, which limits recirculation of the substance after initial injection and allows for multiple ICG angiograms to be done within the same surgical case.[24] Within a neurosurgical case, the surgeon will typically utilize ICG after exposure/dissection of the desired surgical field (Fig. 2A and B). At this time a near infrared laser excitation light source projects on the desired field, ICG bolused by anesthesia into a previously established IV, and an optically filtered camera is used to detect the dye's fluorescence.[25] Advantages over classical angiography include its ease of use and ability to examine the specific surgical field under the magnification of the microscope (visualizing perforators that would be hard to see on unmagnified angiography) and its lack of nephrotoxicity.[26] Angiography, however, remains the gold standard examination of vessel changes; its notable advantages include the ability to see beyond the surgical field, visualization through a bloody field, and consistency through time. Some authors, within the context of aneurysm surgery, have noted a 4% to 21% discordance between the 2 imaging modalities in examination of proper clip placement.[27] One such single-center cohort study noted that ICG angiography led to clip repositioning 8% of the time, a similar rate to prior digital subtraction rates.[28]

Recent advances within ICG fluorescence have allowed for more semiquantitative blood flow examination. The relative fluorescence parameter (FLOW 800, Carl Zeiss Meditec AG, Oberkochen, Germany) analysis of ICG video offers further examination of the blood flow to an examined

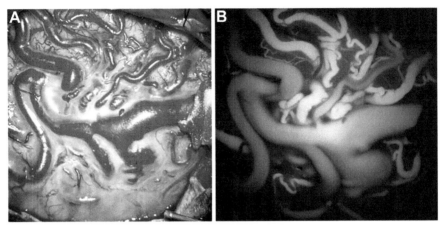

Fig. 2. (A) Microsurgical surface view of the left frontal AVM prior to dissection/resection. (B) ICG angiography of the lesion demonstrating complex vasculature and the course of subarachnoid vessels otherwise difficult to appreciate.

surgical field. This analysis occurs following typical ICG angiography wherein the operating surgeon will select regions of interest (depending on pathology, this includes typically vessels, nidus, or aneurysm) after the ICG video is obtained on the surgical microscope. The relative fluorescence software (a proprietary technology) then measures the intensity of the fluorescence signal garnered from the selected regions of interest. In this manner, each region of interest can generate a relative value of maximum fluorescence, half maximum fluorescence, and time between the two. Furthermore, these values can be graphically compared between regions of interest, offering comparative insight into the surgical field's structures.

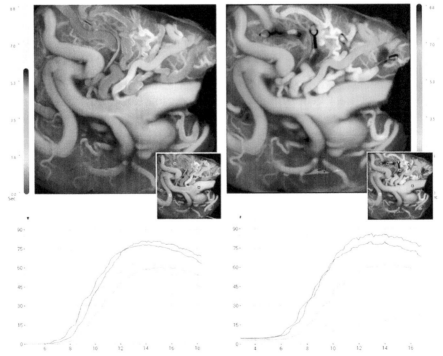

Fig. 3. Relative fluorescence measurements of the left frontal AVM preocclusion and postocclusion of select feeder vessels.

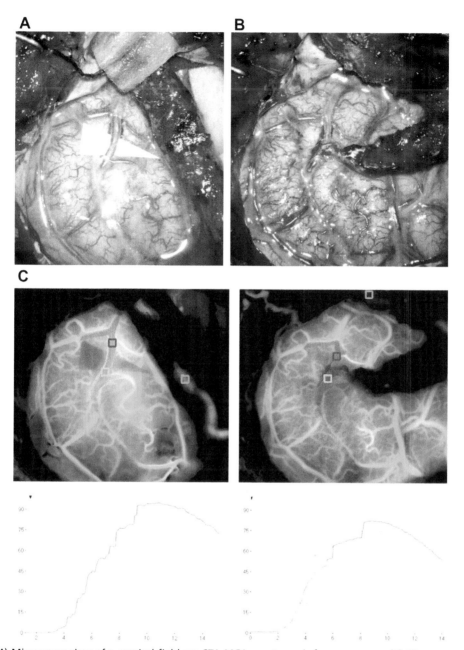

Fig. 4. (*A*) Microscope view of a surgical field pre-STA-MCA anastomosis for moyamoya. (*B*) Microscope view of the cortex after creation of the anastomosis. (*C*) Relative fluorescence measurements of the cortex pre-STA-MCA and post-STA-MCA anastomoses. STA-MCA, superficial temporal artery to middle cerebral artery.

While unable to yield a true quantitative measure such as volumetric flow (cm³/s) or mass transfer (g/s), this remains helpful in pathologies such as AVM, where the relative flow rate of the pathologic nidus and shunt can be compared with more normal neighboring vessels.[29] During open resection, the general flow of artery, vein, and malformation nidus can be examined over time to track progress of the resection (Fig. 3, Videos 1 and 2). Similar utility has been identified in other surgeries as well, and many neurosurgeons continue to find roles for relative fluorescence measurement within their practice.

Many of the studies using relative fluorescence address information gleaned intraoperatively during the open treatment of AVMs, as flow

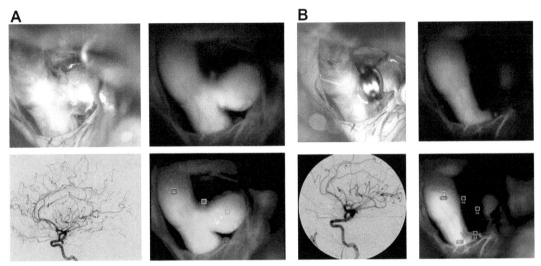

Fig. 5. (*A*) Surgical microscope, DSA, and ICG (angiograph and relative fluorescence) views are shown of a posterior communicating segment aneurysm preclip placement. (*B*) The same microscopic, DSA, and ICG examinations are shown of the aneurysm postclip placement.

dynamics change significantly during the course of the resection. In one study, the mean "transit time" (ie, time to half fluorescence) was prolonged from 0.08 seconds to 2.63 seconds after clipping of AVM feeders, with further prolongation after final nidus resection.[30] Deep AVMs, which can be difficult to visualize from the surface of the brain, can also be more easily identified with relative fluorescence measurement, as the surface vessels will sometimes demonstrated aberrant flow detectable by FLOW 800 despite being grossly normal in appearance to the naked eye.[31] FLOW 800 also offers a semiquantitative way to measure progress of AVM resection by way of examining the major draining vessels. Historically, many have used the color (bright "arterial" red - > dark "venous" red) of prominent draining veins as an informal gage of AVM resection progress; relative fluorescence further describes this process with measures such as transit time and $T_{1/2}$ peak.[32]

Semiquantitative flow measurements have also been described for fistulae and hemangioblastoma resections as well, with one author noting its utility in identifying dominant feeding and draining vessels.[33] FLOW 800 can compare relative fluorescence of multiple sites, making it useful for complex lesions with multiple such entering/egressing vessels, as in dural-AV fistula (dAVF) surgery, where identification of the fistulous point is especially important.[34] Some have also extended this utility in dAVF surgery to the realm of spinal dural AV fistulae.[35] It has also found a home within evaluation of extracranial

to intracranial (EC-IC) bypass, offering insight into hemodynamic changes[36] (**Fig.** 4A–C). In summary, relative fluorescence and time to fluorescence offer useful data regarding hemodynamic changes, even though this technology is unable to give true quantitative measures of flow.

Ultrasound, Doppler, and Other Adjuncts

Advances in ultrasonographic transducer manufacturing have led to applications within neurosurgery. More generally, neurosurgical ultrasonography found its home in oncologic/tumor operations as an adjunct for neuronavigation. Many have found intraoperative ultrasound to be useful, easy to teach, and facile to incorporate in their typical operative workflow.[37] Within the realm of vascular neurosurgery, ultrasound has found a home in efficient localization of intracerebral hemorrhage. Some groups have found that incorporation of surgical ultrasonography in the treatment of hypertensive cerebral hemorrhage lead to more complete hematoma removal, faster procedure times, and better outcomes.[38,39]

Micro-Doppler probes are also used reliably for the evaluation of flow. Classically, micro-Doppler probes found a home in aneurysm surgery as a way to evaluate for complete exclusion of an aneurysm from intravascular flow after clip placement and to evaluate for patency of nearby vessels.[40,41] After placement of a clip, an operating surgeon can gently press the micro-Doppler probe against the structures of interest; the classic "whooshing" pulsatile white-noise sound of moving flow stands

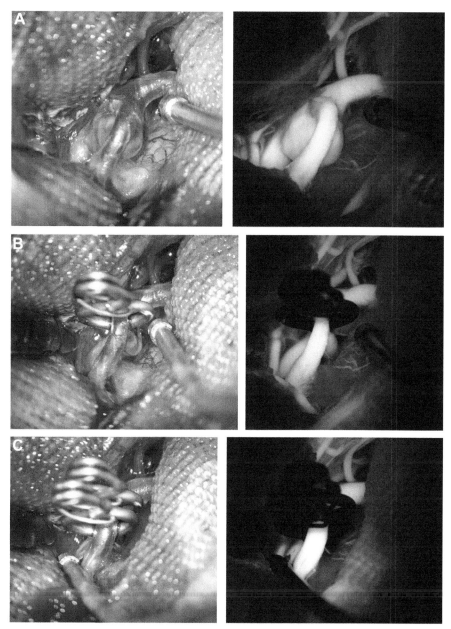

Fig. 6. (A) Microscope and ICG angiography views of a left MCA aneurysm preclipping. (B) Microscope and ICG angiography views of a left MCA aneurysm with 1 clip placed, demonstrating residual aneurysm. (C) Microscope and ICG angiography views of a left MCA aneurysm with 2 clips placed, demonstrating appropriate occlusion of the aneurysm.

in contrast to the frank silence indicated by the absence of flow.

Laser speckle contrast imaging (LSCI) is promising technology in this realm to examine perfusion. LSCI is a wide field optical examination of an operative landscape by analysis of the light speckle interference patterns as perceived by a "charge coupled device," done after illuminating the field with a lens-enhanced laser. In general terms, it offers a way to semiquantitatively examine tissue perfusion,[42] making it a potentially complementary adjunct to relative fluorescence. A recent meta-analysis, however, found limited current use of LSCI in clinical neurosurgery, instead citing works describing preclinical and clinical trial experiences.[43]

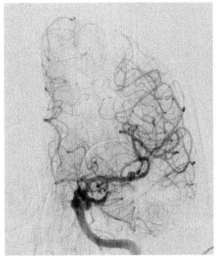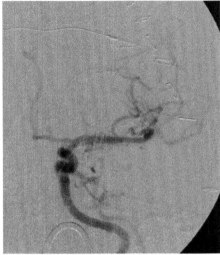

Fig. 7. DSA views (arterial, AP, left carotid injection) of the left MCA aneurysm preclip and postclip application.

SUMMARY

There are many tools available to the vascular neurosurgeon in open cerebrovascular surgery. Traditional DSA remains a familiar staple, and its quality will only improve with the adoption of the hybrid-OR. ICG angiography and its accompanying relative fluorescence analyses offer a powerful way to examine flow within vascular structures and lesions. Ultrasound and associated Doppler technologies represent both the old and the new, with ongoing research on improving its utility as the technology improves to make higher powered ultrasonic transducers. Familiarity with these modalities allows for improved versatility, safety, and efficacy of patient care in the modern age.

CLINICAL CASES
Clinical Case 1

A woman in her early 30s with previous ruptured and coiled anterior communicating artery aneurysm presents in a delayed fashion for microsurgical clipping of a right-sided unruptured posterior communicating artery aneurysm. Fig. 5A and B show microsurgical, angiographic, and ICG (angiographic and relative fluoroscopic) views of the lesion. The postclip application views demonstrate adequate exclusion of the lesion from flow with patency of the parent and adjacently visualized vessels.

Clinical Case 2

A man in his early 50s presents for microsurgical clipping of a left MCA aneurysm. Fig. 6A demonstrates the dissected surgical field and aneurysm prior to clip placement. Fig. 6B demonstrates the lesion after application of 1 fenestrated clip, with

residual indicating unsatisfactory treatment. A second clip was placed, and Fig. 6C demonstrates the final status of the lesion prior to closure. Fig. 7 shows the preoperative angiogram (AP, arterial phase, left carotid injection) of the aneurysm compared with the immediate postclip application intraoperative angiogram.

CLINICS CARE POINTS

- Leaving residual aneurysm during clipping is an undesirable outcome.
- ICG video and/or DSA can demonstrate when clipping of an aneurysm is incomplete and requires further treatment.
- Using intraoperative imaging can guide the surgeon to add another clip, reposition a clip, or change clipping strategy during the surgery.

DISCLOSURES

The authors have nothing to disclose.

SUPPLEMENTARY DATA

Supplementary data related to this article can be found online at https://doi.org/10.1016/j.nic.2024.01.005.

REFERENCES

1. Gruber A, Dorfer C, Standhardt H, et al. Prospective Comparison of Intraoperative Vascular Monitoring

Technologies During Cerebral Aneurysm Surgery. Neurosurgery 2011;68(3):657.

2. Chalouhi N, Theofanis T, Jabbour P, et al. Safety and Efficacy of Intraoperative Angiography in Craniotomies for Cerebral Aneurysms and Arteriovenous Malformations: A Review of 1093 Consecutive Cases. Neurosurgery 2012;71(6):1162.

3. Esposito G, Regli L. Intraoperative tools for cerebral bypass surgery. Acta Neurochir 2018;160(4):775–8.

4. Haranhalli N, Zeberg H, Lasala P, et al. Radiolucent Skull Clamps for Intra-Operative Imaging: A Technical Note. Cureus 2017;9(2):e1020.

5. Kotowski M, Sarrafzadeh A, Schatlo B, et al. Intraoperative angiography reloaded: a new hybrid operating theater for combined endovascular and surgical treatment of cerebral arteriovenous malformations: a pilot study on 25 patients. Acta Neurochir 2013;155(11):2071–8.

6. Barstad RM, Fosse E, Vatne K, et al. Intraoperative Angiography in Minimally Invasive Direct Coronary Artery Bypass Grafting. Ann Thorac Surg 1997; 64(6):1835–9.

7. Gharios M, El-Hajj VG, Frisk H, et al. The use of hybrid operating rooms in neurosurgery, advantages, disadvantages, and future perspectives: a systematic review. Acta Neurochir 2023;165(9): 2343–58.

8. Wang C, Hsu SK, Chang CJ, et al. Transfemoral Approach for Intraoperative Angiography in the Prone or Three-quarter Prone Position : A Revisited Protocol for Intracranial Arteriovenous Malformation and Fistula Surgery. Clin Neuroradiol 2020;30(2): 373–9.

9. Orru' E, Sorte DE, Wolinsky JP, et al. Intraoperative spinal digital subtraction angiography: indications, technique, safety, and clinical impact. J Neurointerventional Surg 2017;9(6):601–7.

10. Villelli NW, Lewis DM, Leipzig TJ, et al. Intraoperative angiography via the popliteal artery: a useful technique for patients in the prone position. J Neurosurg Spine 2018;29(3):322–6.

11. Haynes J, Nossek E, Shapiro M, et al. Radial Arterial Access for Thoracic Intraoperative Spinal Angiography in the Prone Position. World Neurosurg 2020;137:e358–65.

12. Nossek E, Chalif DJ, Buciuc R, et al. Intraoperative Angiography for Arteriovenous Malformation Resection in the Prone and Lateral Positions, Using Upper Extremity Arterial Access. Oper Neurosurg Hagerstown Md 2017;13(3):352–60.

13. Bijlenga P, Mendes Pereira V, Schaller K. Clipping of MCA aneurysms: how I do it. Acta Neurochir 2011; 153(7):1361–6.

14. Payner TD, Horner TG, Leipzig TJ, et al. Role of intraoperative angiography in the surgical treatment of cerebral aneurysms. J Neurosurg 1998;88(3): 441–8.

15. Chiang VL, Gailloud P, Murphy KJ, et al. Routine intraoperative angiography during aneurysm surgery. J Neurosurg 2002;96(6):988–92.

16. Tang G, Cawley CM, Dion JE, et al. Intraoperative angiography during aneurysm surgery: a prospective evaluation of efficacy. J Neurosurg 2002;96(6): 993–9.

17. Martin NA, Bentson J, Viñuela F, et al. Intraoperative digital subtraction angiography and the surgical treatment of intracranial aneurysms and vascular malformations. J Neurosurg 1990;73(4):526–33.

18. Munshi I, Macdonald RL, Weir BKA. Intraoperative Angiography of Brain Arteriovenous Malformations. Neurosurgery 1999;45(3):491.

19. Kato N, Kan I, Abe Y, et al. Visualization of extracranial-intracranial bypass in moyamoya patients using intraoperative three-dimensional digital subtraction angiography with intravenous contrast injection and robotic C-arm: patient series. J Neurosurg Case Lessons 2021;1(4):CASE2057.

20. Tudor T, Sussman J, Sioutas GS, et al. Intraoperative angiography in neurosurgery: temporal trend, access site, and operative indication considerations from a 6-year institutional experience. J Neurointerventional Surg 2023. https://doi.org/10.1136/jnis-2023-020709.

21. Lang SS, Eskioglu E, Mericle R A. Intraoperative angiography for neurovascular disease in the prone or three-quarter prone position. Surg Neurol 2006; 65(3):283–9.

22. Benson RC, Kues HA. Fluorescence properties of indocyanine green as related to angiography. Phys Med Biol 1978;23(1):159.

23. Kogure K, David NJ, Yamanouchi U, et al. Infrared Absorption Angiography of the Fundus Circulation. Arch Ophthalmol 1970;83(2):209–14.

24. Owens SL. Indocyanine green angiography. Br J Ophthalmol 1996;80(3):263–6.

25. Raabe A, Beck J, Gerlach R, et al. Near-infrared Indocyanine Green Video Angiography: A New Method for Intraoperative Assessment of Vascular Flow. Neurosurgery 2003;52(1):132.

26. Świątnicki W, Urbaniak F, Szymański J, et al. Intraoperative fluorescein videoangiography-related nephrotoxicity in intracranial aneurysm surgery: Single center, observational cohort study. Clin Neurol Neurosurg 2021;203:106597.

27. Doss VT, Goyal N, Humphries W, et al. Comparison of Intraoperative Indocyanine Green Angiography and Digital Subtraction Angiography for Clipping of Intracranial Aneurysms. Interv Neurol 2015;3(3–4):129–34.

28. Sharma M, Ambekar S, Ahmed O, et al. The Utility and Limitations of Intraoperative Near-Infrared Indocyanine Green Videoangiography in Aneurysm Surgery. World Neurosurg 2014;82(5):e607–13.

29. Ye X, Liu XJ, Ma L, et al. Clinical values of intraoperative indocyanine green fluorescence video angiography

with Flow 800 software in cerebrovascular surgery. Chin Med J (Engl) 2013;126(22):4232–7.

30. Fukuda K, Kataoka H, Nakajima N, et al. Efficacy of FLOW 800 with Indocyanine Green Videoangiography for the Quantitative Assessment of Flow Dynamics in Cerebral Arteriovenous Malformation Surgery. World Neurosurg 2015;83(2):203–10.

31. Grzyb CC, Church EW. Role of Indocyanine Green with FLOW 800 in Removal of Hidden Arteriovenous Malformations. World Neurosurg 2022;164:e203–13.

32. Zhu J, Chen Z, Zhai W, et al. Non-Angry Superficial Draining Veins: A New Technique in Identifying the Extent of Nidus Excision during Cerebral Arteriovenous Malformation Surgery. Brain Sci 2023;13(2):366.

33. Shah KJ, Cohen-Gadol AA. The Application of FLOW 800 ICG Videoangiography Color Maps for Neurovascular Surgery and Intraoperative Decision Making. World Neurosurg 2019;122:e186–97.

34. Holling M, Brokinkel B, Ewelt C, et al. Dynamic ICG fluorescence provides better intraoperative understanding of arteriovenous fistulae. Neurosurgery 2013;73(1 Suppl Operative). ons:93-98;[discussion ons99].

35. Shi W, Qiao G, Sun Z, et al. Quantitative assessment of hemodynamic changes during spinal dural arteriovenous fistula surgery. J Clin Neurosci Off J Neurosurg Soc Australas 2015;22(7):1155–9.

36. Prinz V, Hecht N, Kato N, et al. FLOW 800 Allows Visualization of Hemodynamic Changes After Extracranial-to-Intracranial Bypass Surgery but Not Assessment of Quantitative Perfusion or Flow. Oper Neurosurg 2014;10(2):231.

37. Dixon L, Lim A, Grech-Sollars M, et al. Camp S. Intraoperative ultrasound in brain tumor surgery: A review and implementation guide. Neurosurg Rev 2022;45(4):2503–15.

38. Gong M, Zhang H, Shi Z, et al. Application of intraoperative ultrasound in neurosurgery for hypertensive intracerebral hemorrhage. J Clin Neurosci Off J Neurosurg Soc Australas 2021;90:251–5.

39. Miao ZL, Jiang L, Xu X, et al. Microsurgical treatment assisted by intraoperative ultrasound localization: a controlled trial in patients with hypertensive basal ganglia hemorrhage. Br J Neurosurg 2014;28(4):478–82.

40. Akdemir H, Oktem IS, Tucer B, et al. Intraoperative microvascular Doppler sonography in aneurysm surgery. Minim Invasive Neurosurg MIN 2006;49(5):312–6.

41. Marchese E, Albanese A, Denaro L, et al. Intraoperative microvascular Doppler in intracranial aneurysm surgery. Surg Neurol 2005;63(4):336–42 [discussion 342].

42. Tao S, Zhang T, Zhou K, et al. Intraoperative Monitoring Cerebral Blood Flow During the Treatment of Brain Arteriovenous Malformations in Hybrid Operating Room by Laser Speckle Contrast Imaging. Front Surg 2022;9:855397.

43. Konovalov A, Gadzhiagaev V, Grebenev F, et al. Laser Speckle Contrast Imaging in Neurosurgery: A Systematic Review. World Neurosurg 2023;171:35–40.

Metabolic Imaging of Acute Ischemic Stroke (PET, ^{1}Hydrogen Spectroscopy, ^{17}Oxygen Imaging, ^{23}Sodium MRI, pH Imaging)

Anil Vasireddi, MD*, Pamela W. Schaefer, MD, Saurabh Rohatgi, MD

KEYWORDS

- Stroke • Metabolic imaging • PET • Hydrogen spectroscopy • MRI • Sodium MRI • pH imaging
- Oxygen imaging

KEY POINTS

- Imaging plays a vital role in management of acute ischemic stroke by estimating areas of benign oligemia, ischemic penumbra and infarct core, which are characterized by differing metabolic derangements.
- A variety of imaging techniques have been tailored to be sensitive to such metabolic derangements, to better characterize the ischemic penumbra. Such information would provide clinicians with insights in refining clinical management and treatment strategies.
- Understanding the unique advantages and limitations associated with each metabolic imaging technique is important to understand their role in clinical application.

INTRODUCTION

Stroke is one of the leading cases of mortality and long-term disability globally.[1,2] Stroke imaging plays a vital role in determining the need for intervention by estimating the ischemic penumbra and brain parenchyma at risk for progression to infarction without acute intervention.

Computed tomography (CT) and magnetic resonance (MR) perfusion techniques are typically used in stroke workflow for the purpose of estimating penumbral volume. Over the past decades, significant strides have been made in accurately differentiating the ischemic penumbra from benign oligemia (oligemic tissue not at risk for infarction) and from the irreversibly infarcted core.

Benign oligemia, ischemic penumbra, and infarct core are characterized by differing cellular responses to diminishing cerebral blood flow (CBF) and thus demonstrate differences in underlying metabolic derangements (Fig. 1). Metabolic imaging offers the potential to provide information at the molecular level to assess tissue viability, refine patient selection for therapy, and guide treatment decisions. This article reviews various metabolic imaging tools including PET, hydrogen (^{1}H) spectroscopy, oxygen-17 (^{17}O) imaging, pH-weighted MRI, and sodium MRI and their role in quantifying various metabolic derangements in acute ischemic stroke.

DISCUSSION
PET Imaging

Multitracer ^{15}O PET

PET imaging with radiotracers containing oxygen-15 (^{15}O) offers a window into the assessment of the impaired oxygen metabolism typical of acute

Division of Neuroradiology, Department of Radiology, Massachusetts General Hospital, Harvard Medical School, 55 Fruit Street, Boston, MA 02114, USA
* Corresponding author.
E-mail address: avasireddi@mgh.harvard.edu

Neuroimag Clin N Am 34 (2024) 271–280
https://doi.org/10.1016/j.nic.2024.01.002

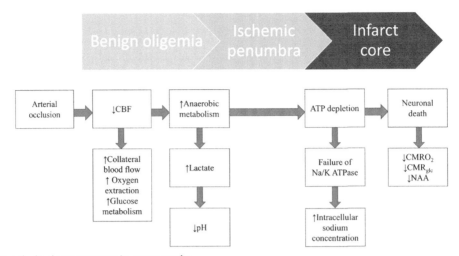

Fig. 1. Metabolic derangements in acute stroke.

ischemic stroke. Measurements of CBF, cerebral blood volume (CBV), mean transit time (MTT), oxygen extraction fraction (OEF) and cerebral metabolic rate of oxygen ($CMRO_2$) can be made with ^{15}O-based PET techniques.[2–7]

The ischemic penumbra refers to the brain parenchyma surrounding the core infarct with decreased CBF resulting in decreased neuronal electrical activity but with otherwise maintained transmembrane electrical potential and ionic homeostasis. ^{15}O PET is particularly useful for the estimation of penumbra in the setting of acute ischemic stroke. PET studies have demonstrated that large volumes of penumbra may persist up to 18 hours after stroke onset, suggesting possible benefit for thrombolysis in patients presenting beyond the conventional therapeutic window of 4.5 hours.[4]

^{15}O PET is usually performed with a combination of multiple oxygen-containing radiotracers with serial PET scans performed after administration of each tracer. These include ^{15}O-oxygen gas (O_2) ($^{15}O_2$) and ^{15}O-carbon monoxide gas (CO) for measurements of CBV and either ^{15}O-carbon dioxide (CO_2) ($C^{15}O_2$) gas or ^{15}O-water (H_2O) ($H_2{}^{15}O$) for measurements of CBF and OEF.[7]

$^{15}O_2$ gas flowing at around 0.5 L/min is inhaled in either a continuous fashion for 8 to 10 minutes or as a bolus for less than 1 minute. PET imaging is subsequently performed to measure kinetics of O_2 metabolism.[7] If administered with continuous inhalation, $C^{15}O_2$ gas is subsequently inhaled and PET imaging is performed for the estimation of CBF. OEF estimation involves division of the $^{15}O_2$ by the $C^{15}O_2$ maps. If $^{15}O_2$ is inhaled via bolus technique instead, PET imaging is performed after intravenous administration of $H_2{}^{15}O$ for estimation of CBF.[7] $CMRO_2$ can also be calculated as a product of CBF, OEF, and arterial blood O_2 concentration.[5]

Finally, PET imaging is performed following inhalation of radiolabeled CO gas for estimation of CBV. Since CO binds irreversibly to hemoglobin, it essentially serves as a blood pool agent.[7] MTT can be calculated as a ratio of CBV divided by CBF.[8]

CBF is progressively diminished in benign oligemia, ischemic penumbra, and infarct core. Areas of completed infarction demonstrate essentially absent CBF (Fig. 2). Diminished cerebral perfusion pressure may also initially result in an elevation in CBV secondary to vasodilation/collateral flow in order to maintain CBF. When vasodilatation is maximal, areas of benign oligemia and ischemic penumbra demonstrate a decrease in CBF and an increase in OEF to preserve $CMRO_2$. These can be differentiated from core infarct, which shows diminished $CMRO_2$.[3,4,8]

^{18}F-Fluorodeoxyglucose PET

Glucose is the primary energy source for brain tissue. Although the brain only makes up 2% of the total body weight, it accounts for 25% of total glucose metabolism.[6] Glucose is transported into neurons and glial cells by a variety of glucose transporter proteins. Intracellularly, glucose is phosphorylated to keep it trapped inside the cell to be further metabolized as a source of energy.[6]

PET imaging to evaluate glucose metabolism can be performed using ^{18}Ffluorodeoxyglucose (FDG), which is also widely used in oncologic assessment. ^{18}F-FDG is administered intravenously and has a much longer half-life of 110 minutes compared to ^{15}O (~2 minutes).[6]

Experimental studies involving stroke models of small animals and primates have shown diminished FDG uptake in the region of the infarct core and elevated ^{18}F-FDG uptake in the

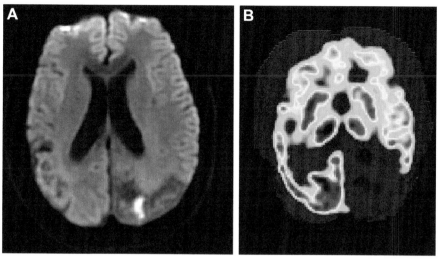

Fig. 2. Diffusion-weighted imaging in a patient with a known history of moyamoya disease shows focal diffusion restriction in the left occipital lobe, corresponding to a subacute infarct superimposed upon an area of encephalomalacia, likely related to an older infarct (*A*). Cerebral blood flow (CBF) map generated with $H_2^{15}O$ PET shows diminished/absent blood flow throughout this region (*B*). (*Courtesy of* G. Zaharchuk, MD, PhD, Stanford University and M. Zhao, PhD, Stanford, CA.)

surrounding penumbra tissue.[6] Sobrado and colleagues[9] showed that ^{18}F-FDG uptake decreases in the acute and early subacute stages after stroke onset in a rat middle cerebral artery occlusion model. Following reperfusion at 24 hours, it was noted that areas that recovered from ischemia demonstrated greater ^{18}F-FDG uptake than those that did not. Animal studies correlating ^{18}FDG-PET with histopathological data similarly showed that areas of completed infarction corresponded to regions of reduced cerebral metabolic rate of glucose (CMR_{glc}) and that the surrounding brain parenchyma which did not progress to infarction demonstrated elevated CMR_{glc}.

Findings suggestive of increased glucose metabolism within the ischemic penumbra have also been demonstrated in human stroke patients[6,9] (Fig. 3). Human data on the use of ^{18}F-FDG-PET in acute stroke remain limited at this time.

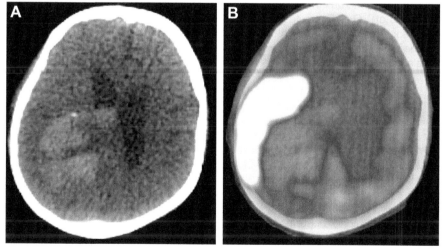

Fig. 3. A 64-year-old male with lymphoma underwent FDG PET for oncologic workup. The patient was found to have an acute right hemispheric infarct with hemorrhagic conversion as shown in non-contrast head CT (*A*). FDG PET demonstrates diminished FDG uptake in the region of the hemorrhage/infarct and markedly increased uptake in the adjacent brain parenchyma (*B*). CT, computed tomography; FDG, fluorodeoxyglucose. (*Adapted from*[35]; with permission.)

Other radiotracers

[11]C-flumazenil (^{11}C-FMZ) and ^{18}F-fluoromisonida-zole (^{18}F-FMISO) are among other PET tracers which have been studied for utility in acute stroke. ^{11}C-FMZ uptake serves as a marker for cortical neuronal integrity.[5] Uptake decreases in irreversibly infarcted tissue. ^{11}C-FMZ PET has been shown to be capable of distinguishing penumbra from core infarct within 3 hours of stroke onset.[4,5] Another benefit with ^{11}C-FMZ is that CBF can be estimated without the need for an arterial blood sample.[5] ^{18}F-FMISO is another agent that binds irreversibly to hypoxic tissue and has been shown to identify hypoxic tissue within 48 hours of stroke onset.[4] However, it has not yet been shown to be reliably capable of differentiating infarct core from penumbra in humans.[10]

There are numerous limitations that currently preclude the use of PET imaging as a standard diagnostic tool in the evaluation of acute ischemic stroke. PET imaging is expensive, not always available, involves the use of ionizing radiation, and often requires complex data analysis following image acquisition.

Long scan times make its use challenging given the time-sensitivity of therapeutic intervention. In addition, long scan times make PET prone to motion/misregistration artifacts with patients who may not always be capable of laying still or following commands. [15]O PET is also particularly challenging given the use of multiple tracers and the complexity of execution with the acquisition of multiple PET scans.

PET capability is also limited by radiotracer availability and the need for the presence of an on-site hot chemistry laboratory due to the relatively short half-lives of positron emitters. In particular, short half-lives of [15]O ($\sim$2 minutes) and [11]C ($\sim$20 minutes) require the presence of an on-site cyclotron for the generation of radiotracers containing these elements.[5]

[1]Hydrogen Spectroscopy

MR spectroscopy (MRS) is a useful tool often used as an ancillary technique to MRI to non-invasively provide information related to tissue chemical composition. Although not typically used in stroke imaging clinically, changes in brain metabolite concentrations in response to ischemia are well characterized in the literature.[11–13]

^{1}H MRS is most commonly performed as the hydrogen nucleus is the most widely prevalent nucleus with a non-zero spin in human tissue and thus provides the highest signal for MRS. The most commonly evaluated ^{1}H MRS metabolites include N-acetylaspartate (NAA), lactate, choline, creatine/phosphocreatine (Cr/PCr), lipids, and myoinositol.[11]

NAA (2.0 ppm) is a marker for neuronal integrity, and decreased NAA is thus associated with neuronal damage/death.[3,11] Lactate (doublet at 1.3 ppm) is a product of and marker for the presence of anaerobic metabolism.[3,13] It is thus a useful marker for the evaluation of ischemic change. Cell membrane degradation results in the release of free fatty acids/lipids yielding multiple peaks around 0.9 to 1.45 ppm.[11] Lipids are thus a marker for tissue necrosis.

Choline (3.2 ppm) is a marker for cell membrane turnover. Cr and PCr are impossible to distinguish spectroscopically (methyl singlet at 3.0 ppm, methylene singlet at 3.9 ppm).[11] They are involved in cellular phosphate transport system and serve as markers for energy metabolism. Myoinositol (3.5 ppm) is a marker of increased glial activity.[12]

Single-slice multi-voxel chemical shift imaging is preferred over single-voxel spectroscopy in acute stroke imaging given its higher spatial resolution and the possible need for interrogation of a large region of ischemia. ^{1}H MRS can be performed simultaneously with conventional stroke protocol MRI. An example of MRS protocol employed in the setting of acute ischemic infarct by Dani and colleagues[13] utilized an echo time (TE) of 144 milliseconds with an approximate sequence duration of 5 minutes.

Acute ischemic stroke has been shown to result in several changes in metabolite concentrations which can be characterized with ^{1}H MRS and reflect the underlying pathology of infarction at the molecular level. NAA and lactate are the 2 most relevant metabolites in acute stroke imaging.[5]

NAA levels have been shown to decrease within the first hour of arterial occlusion, reflecting early loss of neuronal integrity within a developing infarct.[3] MRS studies performed over time in acute ischemic stroke have shown an early rapid decrease in NAA (roughly 20% within 1 hour, 50% within 6 hours in animal models) followed by a more gradual decrease and eventual stabilization by around 1 week.[13]

Animal studies have shown that increases in lactate concentration can be seen within minutes of acute ischemia.[13] Increases in lactate are seen throughout areas of hypoperfusion, extending beyond the infarct core.[11,14] Fig. 4 demonstrates an example of MRS demonstrating elevated lactate in the setting of acute infarct. Lactate concentration can also decrease with reperfusion due to increased clearance.[3,11] Residual lactate signal can persist long after the acute phase.[11]

Changes in NAA and lactate concentrations, as measured by MRS, have been proposed as a potential tool for the identification of tissue at risk

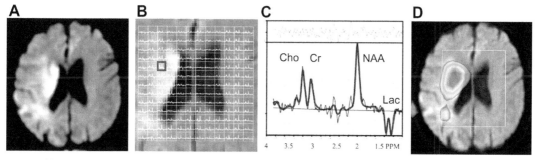

Fig. 4. Diffusion-weighted image shows diffusion restriction in the right caudate nucleus, corona radiata, frontal lobe, and parietal lobe compatible with infarction (*A*). Multivoxel ^{1}H spectroscopy at TE = 135 milliseconds was performed to include the regions of infarction (*B*). MR spectrum from one of the voxels, labeled in red in (*B*), shows a prominent inverted lactate doublet at 1.3 ppm (*C*). A lactate map shows elevated concentrations of lactate corresponding to the regions of DWI hyperintensity (*D*). DWI, diffusion-weighted imaging; MR, magnetic resonance; TE, echo time. (*Courtesy of* E, Ratai, PhD, Boston, MA.)

salvageable with reperfusion.[3,11,13] Cvoro and colleagues[14] characterized metabolite concentrations as measured with MRS in acute ischemic stroke prospectively in a group of 53 patients. Lactate was asymmetrically elevated in all areas in the brain ipsilateral to the location of the infarct compared to normal voxels in the contralateral brain, likely reflecting the effects of oligemia. Although NAA was decreased within the areas of diffusion-weighted imaging (DWI) signal abnormality, no significant difference was identified within penumbral tissue, as defined by a DWI-perfusion-weighted imaging (PWI) mismatch, when compared to the contralateral normal brain. An elevated lactate without decreased NAA may thus be considered as a potential MRS signature for the ischemic penumbra but may also be seen in areas of benign oligemia.

Decreases in Cr/PCr can also be seen in acute ischemic infarct with further decreases seen up to 10 days after the initial ischemic event.[11,15] Choline measurements are variably increased, decreased, or unchanged with ischemia.[11,12,16] Lipids may also increase in the subacute phase with progressive tissue necrosis in the infarct core. These changes are often less apparent than those seen with NAA and lactate.

Prolonged sequence duration, especially with multi-voxel MRS, poses a significant limitation in routine clinical practice in the evaluation of a time-sensitive pathology such as acute ischemic stroke. MRS is also limited by poor signal-to-noise ratio (SNR), complexity of the acquisition techniques with multi-voxel MRS, suboptimal spatial resolution, and the risk of lipid contamination with motion. Overlap in signals from different metabolites sharing similar resonant frequencies (eg, lactate and lipids) can also make differentiation challenging.

^{17}Oxygen Imaging

^{17}O MRS offers an approach to measuring oxygen consumption alternative to ^{15}O PET. ^{17}O is among the 3 stable isotopes of oxygen (others being the ^{16}O and ^{18}O) and is the only one that can be detected by MR.[16]

The vast majority of measured signal in ^{17}O MRS is derived from oxygen in water molecules.[16] ^{17}O$_2$ gas is inhaled, absorbed into tissues, and eventually incorporated into water molecules as part of normal cellular respiration. Rate of H$_2$^{17}O production is thought to reflect the cellular metabolic rate of oxygen.

CBF can be estimated either via monitoring washout kinetics of exogenous H$_2$^{17}O administered intraarterially or intravenously. Alternatively, a methodology has also been developed to noninvasively measure CBF by monitoring signal from endogenous H$_2$^{17}O generated within the mitochondria following inhalation of ^{17}O$_2$ gas. Quantitative measurements of OEF can also be calculated with the following equation: OEF = CMRO$_2$/(arterial oxygen concentration × CBF).[16]

^{17}O MRS has been tested in preclinical animal models of ischemic stroke at field strengths ranging from 3T to 16.4 T.[16,17] Feasibility studies have also been performed in humans allowing for noninvasive simultaneous measurements of CMRO$_2$, CBF, and OEF after ^{17}O$_2$ inhalation.[16,17] However, additional studies are needed for further characterization of imaging findings in acute ischemic stroke in human subjects.

Application of ^{17}O MRS in routine clinical practice is limited by a number of factors. Translation to human subjects requires a better understanding of ^{17}O kinetics in humans compared to small animal models.[3,16] ^{17}O has lower detection sensitivity for MR than ^{1}H and may require high-field systems to maintain SNR. As with most MRS techniques, spatial resolution is another limitation. Cost is another potential hurdle for clinical application as [17]O-enriched gas is highly expensive due to its limited supply.[16]

[23]Sodium MRI

Sodium MRI relies on MR signal obtained from the [23]Na nucleus. [23]Na is found in all living cells and is the second most abundantly detected element in the human body after [1]H. MR signal derived from [23]Na is roughly 10,000 less than that of [1]H.[18]

Sodium plays many important roles in normal cellular function including osmoregulation, pH regulation, and maintaining a transmembrane electrochemical gradient necessary for the propagation of action potentials in neurons and muscle cells.[19] This gradient is established by a sodium-potassium adenosinetriphosphatase (ATPase) channel, which exports sodium ions from and imports potassium ions into the cell.

Sodium MRI can provide a measure of total sodium concentration (TSC) as a volume-weighted average of intracellular sodium concentration (ISC) and extracellular sodium concentration (ESC). In pathologies of cellular energy deficiency, such as acute stroke, failure of normal sodium-potassium ATPase function results in a net influx of sodium ions into the cell (Fig. 5). Although ISC markedly increases, ESC is buffered by the body and is less affected. This results in an overall increase in TSC, which has been demonstrated both in animal stroke models and also clinically in human patients.[20,21]

The inherently low signal derived from [23]Na nuclei, which is orders of magnitude lower than that derived from ^{1}H, is a major limitation of sodium MRI.[18] Rapid decay of transverse magnetization after each radiofrequency pulse further limits SNR.[19] These challenges of sodium MRI demand imaging techniques that maximize SNR including imaging with a high field strength, a very short TE (<1 millisecond), multiple measurements, and large voxel sizes, yielding long scan times and low spatial resolution.[18,22,23] Scan times of approximately 6 minutes have been described in the literature performed in the setting of acute ischemic stroke.[22,23]

Resonant frequency of sodium nuclei also differs from hydrogen. Radiofrequency coils capable of transmitting and detecting MR signal from sodium nuclei are thus necessary. Such coils may be single tuned to sodium signal or dual tuned and capable of acquiring signal from sodium and hydrogen.[19] In the case of single-tuned coils, coils may either have to be swapped between proton and sodium MR acquisitions or the patient may need to be transported between scanners, further adding to the total scan time.

TSC in normal brain parenchyma has been reported in the range of 30 to 56 mM, with values slightly higher in gray matter compared to white matter.[18,20] TSC in cerebrospinal fluid (CSF) is significantly higher and equivalent to ESC (~140 mM) and can result in artifactual elevations in TSC from partial volume effects.[20]

The key imaging feature of sodium MRI in acute ischemic stroke is a time-dependent increase in TSC within the region of infarction. Changes in TSC within the region of infarction defined by DWI signal abnormality can be minimal (<10%) within the first 7 hours of infarction.[22] This is followed by a more rapid increase with a somewhat linear rate of increase measuring ~2% per hour.[21] TSC then begins to plateau around 48 hours.[22] Fig. 6 shows an example of elevated TSC using sodium MRI, which corresponds to a

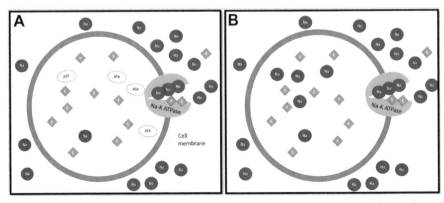

Fig. 5. Sodium-potassium adenosinetriphosphatase (ATPase) maintains normal electrochemical gradient across the cell membrane by importing 2 potassium ions and exporting 3 sodium ions at the cost of 1 ATP molecule (A). Loss of transport function upon ATP depletion results in progressive increase in intracellular sodium concentration and loss of the normal electrical membrane gradient (B). ATP, adenosine triphosphate.

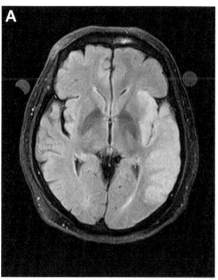
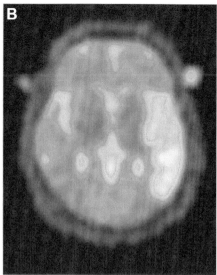

Fig. 6. T2-weighted fluid-attenuated inversion recovery (FLAIR) image with standard ¹H MRI shows hyperintensity in the left temporal lobe and insular corresponding to an middle cerebral artery (MCA) distribution infarct (A). ²³Na MRI demonstrates elevated total sodium concentration (TSC) in the region of signal abnormality (B). (*Adapted from*[24]; with permission.)

region of T2 FLAIR signal abnormality on proton MRI.[24]

There is also regional variability in rates of TSC increase in acute infarction. Primate studies have demonstrated that rates of increase are greatest centrally within the infarct core and lower peripherally.[20] Rate of increase in TSC may also depend on location of the infarct. Infarcts in the basal ganglia tend to have more rapid increases in TSC compared to the cortex, which may reflect relative paucity of collateral flow to the basal ganglia.[20]

In contrast to the core infarct, increases in TSC are less apparent within the penumbra. In fact, animal studies have shown a slight decrease in TSC within penumbra tissue in the acute stage (as defined by presence of a DWI-PWI mismatch), which may be related to shift of water into the intracellular compartment and associated increases and decreases in contributions of ISC and ESC, respectively, to the TSC.[21,25] This finding has not been demonstrated in human studies, which have shown that TSC does not significantly change in penumbral tissue.[23]

These findings suggest utility of sodium MRI in selecting patients for reperfusion therapy, especially among those who present after 4.5 hours of symptom onset. Absence of any increase in TSC within the area of PWI-DWI mismatch compared to the contralateral brain suggests the presence of salvageable tissue at risk and the potential benefit for reperfusion. A TSC of 70 mM/L compared to the contralateral homologous brain parenchyma has also been suggested as a marker

for a completed infarct based on animal studies comparing imaging and histopathological data although actual values for the threshold are thought to be even lower.[23]

Given the monophasic increase in TSC with time after stroke onset in the acute phase, another potential application of sodium MRI is the estimation of stroke onset time in patients presenting with wake-up strokes. This remains a work in progress as animal studies have yielded variable results in accurately estimating stroke onset times by retrospective linear extrapolation of data from sodium MRI.[21]

pH Imaging

Changes in tissue pH are among the early metabolic derangements that occur during ischemia within penumbral tissue before it proceeds to infarction.[2] Capability to image tissue pH therefore offers an opportunity to better discriminate benign oligemia from penumbra within areas of reduced CBF.

Hypoxemia and energy demands necessitate an increase in anaerobic glycolysis to generate adenosine triphosphate, resulting in a buildup of lactate and tissue acidosis. An increase in partial pressure carbon dioxide also contributes to this acidosis.[26] Normal intracellular pH level usually rests around 7.2. In animal stroke models, tissue pH has been shown to range from 6.5 to 6.9 within the penumbra and as low as 6.0 within the infarct core.[26]

³¹P MRS is considered the gold standard for the noninvasive estimation of tissue pH in vivo.[26] The

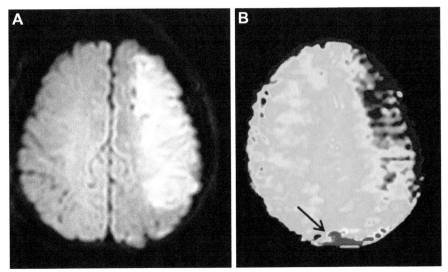

Fig. 7. Diffusion-weighted image shows restricted diffusion in the left middle cerebral artery distribution (*A*). Amide proton transfer (APT)–weighted image shows low signal in the area corresponding to the infarct bed, corresponding to decreased pH (*B*). Note the presence of artifact related to cerebrospinal fluid (*black arrow*). (*Courtesy of* Jinyuan Zhou, PhD, Baltimore, MD, USA, and Min Chen, MD, Beijing, China.[31])

peak corresponding to signal from inorganic phosphate (P_i) experiences a chemical shift that is dependent on pH, while other phosphorus-containing compounds are relatively unaffected. Thus, intracellular pH can be estimated by measuring the chemical shift between the P_i and PCr peaks.[26]

MRS is limited by poor spatial resolution and temporal resolution. In addition, ^{31}P MRS is also limited by poor SNR due to relatively lower natural abundance and lower gyromagnetic ratio of ^{31}P compared to ^1H, necessitating use of high-field MRI and prolonged acquisition times.[26] The use

of specialized MR coils sensitive to signal from ^{31}P additionally makes this technique challenging.

Amide proton transfer (APT) MRI offers an alternative method for noninvasive imaging of tissue pH. APT MRI relies on chemical exchange saturation transfer (CEST) effects, which are sensitive to the presence of functional groups, such as amides, amines, and hydroxyl groups. These groups participate in exchange of protons with water upon application of a radiofrequency pulse at their specific resonance, which results in a decrease in signal obtained from hydrogen atoms in water.[26–28]

Table 1
Metabolic imaging findings of acute stroke

Imaging Technique	Benign Oligemia	Ischemic Penumbra	Infarct Core
PET	↓CBF ↑or normal OEF	↓↓CBF ↑OEF ↑CMR_{glc}	↓↓↓CBF Variable OEF ↓$CMRO_2$ ↓CMR_{glu}
^{1}Hydrogen magnetic resonance spectroscopy (^1H MRS)	↑ or normal lactate	↑Lactate	↑Lactate ↓NAA
^{17}Oxygen magnetic resonance spectroscopy (^{17}O MRS)	↓CBF ↑ or normal OEF	↓↓CBF ↑OEF	↓↓↓CBF Variable OEF ↓$CMRO_2$
^{23}Sodium MRI (^{23}Na MRI)	Normal	Normal	↑TSC
pH MRI	Normal	↓pH	↓↓pH

Abbreviations: CBF, cerebral blood flow; CMR_{glc}, cerebral metabolic rate of glucose; $CMRO_2$, cerebral metabolic rate of oxygen; NAA, N-acetylaspartate; OEF, oxygen extraction fraction; TSC, total sodium concentration.

The exchange between water and amide groups is base catalyzed. As tissue becomes more acidotic in ischemia, the rate of exchange also decreases and amide contribution to the CEST effects becomes less prominent, allowing for mapping of tissue pH. pH would be expected to be normal in normal brain tissue and areas of benign oligemia and progressively reduced in penumbra and core infarct[28–30] (Fig. 7). Serial APT MRI examinations have shown that the decrease in pH associated with infarct can be detectable in the hyperacute stage and tissue acidification can improve in the subacute phase.[31]

APT MRI provides better spatial resolution and SNR with much shorter scan times compared to ^{31}P MRS.[26] Heo and colleagues[32] demonstrated feasibility of APT MRI on a 3T magnet in acute stroke patients with a scan time of 3.2 minutes. It has shown promise for clinical application in differentiating the areas of perfusion and diffusion mismatch into true penumbra and benign oligemia, showing potential as a complementary tool to conventional MRI techniques in stroke.[29,33] The addition of pH-weighted imaging data has also been shown to improve prediction of tissue outcome compared with perfusion-diffusion mismatch data alone.[34]

Like Na MRI, pH-weighted MRI is also susceptible to artifacts from CSF. However, it does not require specialized coils or high magnetic fields. pH-weighted imaging with APT MRI remains understudied in humans and additional experiments are necessary to better characterize the imaging findings in acute ischemic stroke.

SUMMARY

Identification of penumbral tissue has been at the forefront of stroke imaging research over many decades. The use of metabolic imaging techniques to more directly evaluate the metabolic derangements underlying acute stroke (as summarized in Table 1) can provide information complementary to that available with standard CT and MR techniques to more accurately estimate volume of tissue at risk for acute infarction, help direct management decisions, and improve patient outcomes.

CLINICS CARE POINTS

- PET imaging: [15]O PET has been shown to be useful in the estimation of penumbra. Expense, limited availability, longer scan times, radiotracer availability and use of additional anatomical imaging techniques limit its use in acute stroke setting.

- [1]H spectroscopy: Widely available and can be combined with existing MR techniques to help narrow the differential diagnosis. Scan times, low spatial resolution and artifact limit its use.

- [17]O imaging: Mostly still in the research realm with further large-scale studies in human subjects still needing validation. Low resolution, cost and technical challenges limit its application.

- [23]Sodium MRI: Useful as a surrogate marker for tissue viability and could complement conventional CT and MR techniques in selecting patients for reperfusion therapy. Low signal to noise ratio, specialized coils and long scan times limit utility of sodium MRI in acute settings.

- pH imaging: APT MRI is a promising methodology in generating pH weighted MR images, potentially capable of differentiating penumbra from benign oligemia. Low resolution images and technical challenges limit clinical application.

DISCLOSURE

The authors have nothing to disclose.

REFERENCES

1. Collaborators GBDS. Global, regional, and national burden of stroke and its risk factors, 1990-2019: a systematic analysis for the Global Burden of Disease Study 2019. Lancet Neurol 2021;20(10): 795–820.
2. Wey HY, Desai VR, Duong TQ. A review of current imaging methods used in stroke research. Neurol Res 2013;35(10):1092–102.
3. Dani KA, Warach S. Metabolic imaging of ischemic stroke: the present and future. AJNR Am J Neuroradiol 2014;35(6 Suppl):S37–43.
4. Ermine CM, Bivard A, Parsons MW, et al. The ischemic penumbra: From concept to reality. Int J Stroke 2021;16(5):497–509.
5. Lu J, Mei Q, Hou X, et al. Imaging Acute Stroke: From One-Size-Fit-All to Biomarkers. Front Neurol 2021;12:697779.
6. Bunevicius A, Yuan H, Lin W. The potential roles of 18F-FDG-PET in management of acute stroke patients. BioMed Res Int 2013;2013:634598.
7. Fan AP, An H, Moradi F, et al. Quantification of brain oxygen extraction and metabolism with [(15)O]-gas PET: A technical review in the era of PET/MRI. Neuroimage 2020;220:117136.
8. González RG. Acute ischemic stroke : imaging and intervention. Berlin, Heidelberg: Springer; 2005. p. 268, xii.

9. Sobrado M, Delgado M, Fernandez-Valle E, et al. Longitudinal studies of ischemic penumbra by using 18F-FDG PET and MRI techniques in permanent and transient focal cerebral ischemia in rats. Neuroimage 2011;57(1):45–54.

10. Alawneh JA, Moustafa RR, Marrapu ST, et al. Diffusion and perfusion correlates of the 18F-MISO PET lesion in acute stroke: pilot study. Eur J Nucl Med Mol Imaging 2014;41(4):736–44.

11. Saunders DE. MR spectroscopy in stroke. Br Med Bull 2000;56(2):334–45.

12. Mazibuko N, Tuura RO, Sztriha L, et al. Subacute Changes in N-Acetylaspartate (NAA) Following Ischemic Stroke: A Serial MR Spectroscopy Pilot Study. Diagnostics 2020;10(7).

13. Dani KA, An L, Henning EC, et al. Multivoxel MR spectroscopy in acute ischemic stroke: comparison to the stroke protocol MRI. Stroke 2012;43(11): 2962–7.

14. Cvoro V, Marshall I, Armitage PA, et al. MR diffusion and perfusion parameters: relationship to metabolites in acute ischaemic stroke. J Neurol Neurosurg Psychiatry 2010;81(2):185–91.

15. Walker PM, Ben Salem D, Lalande A, et al. Time course of NAA T2 and ADC(w) in ischaemic stroke patients: 1H MRS imaging and diffusion-weighted MRI. J Neurol Sci 2004;220(1–2):23–8.

16. Zhu XH, Chen W. In vivo(17)O MRS imaging - Quantitative assessment of regional oxygen consumption and perfusion rates in living brain. Anal Biochem 2017;529:171–8.

17. Zhu XH, Lu M, Chen W. Quantitative imaging of brain energy metabolisms and neuroenergetics using in vivo X-nuclear (2)H, (17)O and (31)P MRS at ultra-high field. J Magn Reson 2018;292:155–70.

18. Hagiwara A, Bydder M, Oughourlian TC, et al. Sodium MR Neuroimaging. AJNR Am J Neuroradiol 2021;42(11):1920–6.

19. Madelin G, Regatte RR. Biomedical applications of sodium MRI in vivo. J Magn Reson Imaging 2013; 38(3):511–29.

20. Thulborn KR, Davis D, Snyder J, et al. Sodium MR imaging of acute and subacute stroke for assessment of tissue viability. Neuroimaging Clin N Am 2005;15(3):639–53. xi-xii.

21. Wetterling F, Gallagher L, Mullin J, et al. Sodium-23 magnetic resonance imaging has potential for improving penumbra detection but not for estimating stroke onset time. J Cereb Blood Flow Metab 2015; 35(1):103–10.

22. Hussain MS, Stobbe RW, Bhagat YA, et al. Sodium imaging intensity increases with time after human ischemic stroke. Ann Neurol 2009;66(1):55–62.

23. Tsang A, Stobbe RW, Asdaghi N, et al. Relationship between sodium intensity and perfusion deficits in acute ischemic stroke. J Magn Reson Imaging 2011;33(1):41–7.

24. Adlung A, Licht C, Reichert S, et al. Quantification of tissue sodium concentration in the ischemic stroke: A comparison between external and internal references for (23)Na MRI. J Neurosci Methods 2022; 382:109721.

25. Wetterling F, Chatzikonstantinou E, Tritschler L, et al. Investigating potentially salvageable penumbra tissue in an in vivo model of transient ischemic stroke using sodium, diffusion, and perfusion magnetic resonance imaging. BMC Neurosci 2016;17(1):82.

26. Larkin JR, Foo LS, Sutherland BA, et al. Magnetic Resonance pH Imaging in Stroke - Combining the Old With the New. Front Physiol 2021;12:793741.

27. Sun PZ. Quasi-steady-state amide proton transfer (QUASS APT) MRI enhances pH-weighted imaging of acute stroke. Magn Reson Med 2022;88(6): 2633–44.

28. Wu Y, Zhou IY, Lu D, et al. pH-sensitive amide proton transfer effect dominates the magnetization transfer asymmetry contrast during acute ischemia-quantification of multipool contribution to in vivo CEST MRI. Magn Reson Med 2018;79(3):1602–8.

29. Cheung J, Doerr M, Hu R, et al. Refined Ischemic Penumbra Imaging with Tissue pH and Diffusion Kurtosis Magnetic Resonance Imaging. Transl Stroke Res 2021;12(5):742–53.

30. Tee YK, Harston GW, Blockley N, et al. Comparing different analysis methods for quantifying the MRI amide proton transfer (APT) effect in hyperacute stroke patients. NMR Biomed 2014;27(9):1019–29.

31. Song G, Li C, Luo X, et al. Evolution of Cerebral Ischemia Assessed by Amide Proton Transfer-Weighted MRI. Front Neurol 2017;8:67.

32. Heo HY, Zhang Y, Burton TM, et al. Improving the detection sensitivity of pH-weighted amide proton transfer MRI in acute stroke patients using extrapolated semisolid magnetization transfer reference signals. Magn Reson Med 2017;78(3):871–80.

33. Tietze A, Blicher J, Mikkelsen IK, et al. Assessment of ischemic penumbra in patients with hyperacute stroke using amide proton transfer (APT) chemical exchange saturation transfer (CEST) MRI. NMR Biomed 2014;27(2):163–74.

34. Jokivarsi KT, Hiltunen Y, Tuunanen PI, et al. Correlating tissue outcome with quantitative multiparametric MRI of acute cerebral ischemia in rats. J Cereb Blood Flow Metab 2010;30(2):415–27.

35. Dundar A, Bold MS, Agac B, et al. Stroke detection with 3 different PET tracers. Radiol Case Rep 2019; 14(11):1447–51.

Vessel Wall Characterization Using Quantitative MR Imaging

Joseph J. Gemmete, MD, FACR, FSIR, FCIRSE, FAHA

KEYWORDS

- 2D black-blood MR imaging • 3D black blood MR imaging
- Dynamic contrast-enhanced magnetic resonance (DCE-MR) imaging
- Flow-derived biomechanical wall parameters • T1 and T2 relaxometry

KEY POINTS

- Two-dimensional and three-dimensional black-blood MR imaging is valuable in identifying and quantifying various plaque components such as the fibrous cap, lipid core, and calcifications.
- MR imaging relaxometry, involving T1 and T2 relaxation time measurements, is a powerful tool in the characterization of atherosclerotic plaque composition.
- Diffusion-weighted imaging can provide information about the cellular composition of the plaque, particularly the presence of a high-density macrophage population, which is often associated with inflammation and plaque instability.
- Dynamic contrast-enhanced MR imaging helps in identifying high-risk plaques, thus aiding in the risk stratification of patients.
- Biomechanical properties such as wall shear stress and arterial stiffness can be measured with MR imaging techniques and play a role in plaque formation and progression and maybe a marker of cardiovascular risk and aging.

INTRODUCTION

The intricate characterization of vessel walls is a cornerstone in understanding and managing vascular diseases, particularly atherosclerosis. MR imaging has revolutionized this domain by providing a noninvasive window into the vascular system, surpassing traditional imaging methods in both safety and efficacy. This article focuses on the comprehensive analysis of vessel wall characterization using various quantitative MR imaging techniques, underscoring their pivotal role in diagnosing and monitoring vascular pathologies.

MR imaging's unparalleled ability to visualize and quantify different aspects of the vessel wall, including plaque burden, composition, and biomechanical properties, offers a unique advantage in the field of vascular imaging. By employing techniques like two-dimensional (2D) and three-dimensional (3D) black-blood MR imaging, T1 and T2 relaxometry, diffusion-weighted imaging (DWI), and dynamic contrast-enhanced MR (DCE-MR) imaging, clinicians and researchers can gain in-depth insights into the nature and progression of vascular diseases.

The importance of this topic lies not only in the academic pursuit of understanding vascular pathology but also in its practical implications for patient care. Accurate vessel wall characterization can guide therapeutic decisions, monitor treatment

Department of Radiology, Michigan Medicine, 1500 East Medical Center Drive, UH B1D 328, Ann Arbor, MI 48109

E-mail addresses: gemmete@med.umich.edu; interventionalist13@gmail.com

Twitter: @joeyg132513 (J.J.G.)

Neuroimag Clin N Am 34 (2024) 281–292

https://doi.org/10.1016/j.nic.2024.02.002

efficacy, and predict clinical outcomes. Thus, this article aims to provide a comprehensive overview of the current state of vessel wall imaging using MR imaging, emphasizing its clinical relevance, technical advancements, and future potential.

ROLE OF MR IMAGING IN ASSESSING PLAQUE BURDEN

MR imaging has emerged as a sophisticated tool in the evaluation of plaque burden. Unlike traditional luminal imaging techniques, MR imaging provides a detailed view of the vessel wall itself, enabling the assessment of both the size and composition of atherosclerotic plaques.[1] With its excellent soft tissue contrast, MR imaging can differentiate between various components of the plaque, such as the fibrous cap, lipid core, and calcifications.[2] This capability is crucial in identifying vulnerable plaques that are at a higher risk of rupture.[3]

Advanced MR imaging techniques, such as high-resolution black-blood MR imaging, have significantly enhanced our ability to visualize small plaques that were previously undetectable with other imaging modalities. Black-blood MR imaging techniques suppress the signal from blood, providing a clear view of the vessel wall and plaques. This is particularly important in coronary artery imaging, where the small size of the arteries and the motion due to heartbeat pose significant challenges.[4]

Furthermore, MR imaging does not involve ionizing radiation, making it a safer option for patients, especially when repeated examinations are required. This aspect is particularly pertinent in longitudinal studies where plaque progression is monitored over time.

Advantages of MR Imaging over Other Imaging Modalities

The advantages of MR imaging over other imaging modalities in assessing plaque burden are multifaceted. First, its superior soft tissue contrast allows for a more detailed characterization of plaque components compared to computed tomography (CT) or ultrasound.[5] While CT is excellent for detecting calcifications, it is less effective in identifying noncalcified plaque components. MR imaging, on the other hand, can differentiate between fibrous, lipid-rich, and calcified components within the plaque.

Second, MR imaging is limited neither by the acoustic window nor by calcification shadowing issues that can hamper ultrasound imaging. This makes MR imaging more reliable for comprehensive plaque assessment, particularly in regions difficult to image with ultrasound, such as the carotid artery bifurcation or the aortic arch.

Third, MR imaging's noninvasive nature and lack of ionizing radiation make it an ideal choice for repeated measurements, which is essential for monitoring disease progression or the response to therapy. This is a significant advantage over CT, which, despite its high resolution, involves exposure to ionizing radiation.

Lastly, MR imaging provides functional information, such as plaque perfusion and vessel wall edema, through techniques like DCE-MR and T2-weighted imaging. This functional assessment is vital for understanding the biological activity of the plaque, which cannot be adequately assessed by CT or ultrasound.

In conclusion, MR imaging represents a comprehensive tool for the assessment of plaque burden in vascular disease. Its ability to provide detailed anatomic and functional information, coupled with its safety profile, makes it an invaluable modality in the diagnosis, risk stratification, and management of patients with atherosclerotic disease. As MR imaging technology continues to advance, its role in understanding and managing vascular pathology is expected to grow further, offering new avenues for research and clinical practice.

TWO-DIMENSIONAL BLACK-BLOOD MR IMAGING
Technical Principles of 2D Black-Blood MR Imaging

Two-dimensional black-blood MR imaging is a specialized MR imaging technique designed to enhance the visibility of blood vessel walls and surrounding tissues by suppressing the signal from flowing blood. This technique is crucial in vascular imaging, particularly for characterizing atherosclerotic plaque within the vessel walls (Fig. 1).

The primary mechanism behind black-blood MR imaging is the use of prepulse sequences that null the signal from flowing blood. This is typically achieved through 2 methods: double inversion recovery and spatial presaturation.[6–8] In double inversion recovery, 2 inversion pulses are applied. The first inverts the magnetization of all tissues, while the second selectively reinverts the static tissue, leaving the blood with a low signal. In spatial presaturation, saturation pulses are applied upstream of the imaging slice, effectively nulling the signal of incoming blood. These spatial saturation pulses are followed by strong spoiled gradients along the phase encoding and frequency encoding axes resulting in further suppression of residual transverse magnetization.

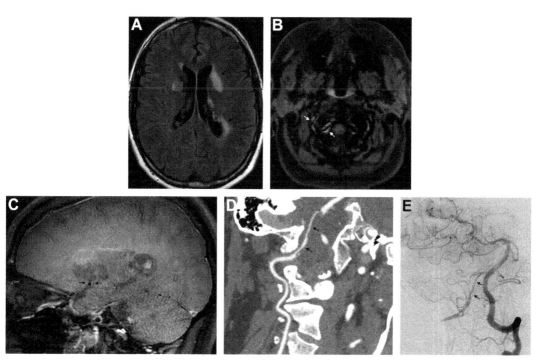

Fig. 1. (A) Axial FLAIR MR imaging of the brain shows abnormal high signal within the left basal ganglia and periventricular white matter (black arrows). (B and C) Two-dimensional black-blood MR imaging shows abnormal enhancement of the vessel wall involving the V3 and V4 segments of the vertebral artery (white arrows) and middle cerebral artery within the sylvian fissure (black arrows). (D) Corresponding MIP CTA image of the right vertebral artery shows an area of narrowing corresponding to the black-blood MR images (black arrows). (E) Oblique left vertebral arteriogram shows narrowing of the V3 and V4 segment of the right vertebral artery (black arrows) corresponding to the findings on the CTA and MR imaging. (A 55 year old woman presented with right-sided weakness and dizziness. She was later diagnosed with a medium arterial size vasculitis.)

These techniques result in images where the blood appears dark ("black-blood"), in contrast to the vessel wall and plaque components, which retain higher signal intensity. This contrast allows for precise delineation of the vessel wall boundaries and detailed characterization of the plaque morphology.

Applications in Plaque Characterization

Two-dimensional black-blood MR imaging is extensively used for the characterization of atherosclerotic plaque.[9] Its ability to provide high-resolution images of the vessel wall makes it particularly valuable in identifying and quantifying various plaque components such as the fibrous cap, lipid core, and calcifications. By differentiating these components, 2D black-blood MR imaging plays a pivotal role in assessing plaque stability and the risk of rupture, which are essential factors in managing cardiovascular risk in patients.[10]

This technique is particularly effective in carotid artery imaging, where it can identify high-risk features of carotid plaques, such as intraplaque

hemorrhage or a thin or ruptured fibrous cap. These features are critical markers of stroke risk, and their identification can influence clinical management strategies, including decisions regarding surgical intervention.[11]

Moreover, 2D black-blood MR imaging is useful in serial imaging to monitor plaque progression or regression over time.[12] This is particularly important in clinical trials and studies assessing the efficacy of various therapeutic interventions on plaque burden and composition.

Limitations and Potential Pitfalls

While 2D black-blood MR imaging offers significant advantages in plaque characterization, it is not without limitations and potential pitfalls. One major limitation is the slice-by-slice acquisition approach, which can be time-consuming and may lead to misregistration errors. This is particularly problematic in areas subject to motion, such as the thoracic and abdominal regions.

Another challenge is the limited coverage area of 2D imaging. Comprehensive assessment of long vessel segments, such as the entire carotid artery, can be time-consuming and may require multiple imaging sessions, which can be impractical in clinical settings.

The spatial resolution, although high, may still be insufficient either to detect very small plaques or to fully characterize plaque components with high precision. This limitation can potentially lead to underestimation of plaque burden or misclassification of plaque type.

Additionally, 2D black-blood MR imaging may suffer from signal-to-noise ratio limitations, particularly in low-field scanners. This can affect image quality and the ability to distinguish between different plaque components accurately.

Lastly, patient-specific factors, such as high heart rates or irregular breathing, can affect image quality. Motion artifacts, in particular, can lead to diagnostic challenges and require careful patient preparation and potentially the use of motion correction techniques during the imaging process.[13]

In conclusion, while 2D black-blood MR imaging is a powerful tool for plaque characterization in vascular imaging, its limitations must be acknowledged. Understanding these limitations is essential for accurate interpretation of imaging findings and for guiding clinical decision-making. Future advancements in MR imaging technology, including higher resolution imaging and improved motion correction techniques, are likely to enhance the utility of this technique in clinical practice.

THREE-DIMENSIONAL BLACK-BLOOD MR IMAGING
Advancements in 3D Black-Blood MR Imaging

Three-dimensional black-blood MR imaging represents a significant advancement in the field of vascular imaging, offering comprehensive and detailed visualization of vessel walls and atherosclerotic plaques. This technique builds on the principles of traditional 2D black-blood MR imaging but extends its capabilities through 3D volumetric imaging, allowing for the acquisition of data in a contiguous block rather than individual slices.[14]

One of the key advancements in 3D black-blood MR imaging is the use of improved pulse sequences and magnetization-prepared rapid gradient-echo sequences.[15–17] These technical enhancements facilitate better blood signal suppression, higher spatial resolution, and reduced motion artifacts. Additionally, developments in parallel imaging and compressed sensing have significantly accelerated data acquisition, making 3D black-blood MR imaging more feasible and patient-friendly.[18]

Recent iterations of 3D black-blood MR imaging also incorporate advanced techniques such as motion-sensitized driven equilibrium preparation, which further suppresses the blood signal and enhances the contrast between the vessel wall and lumen.[19,20] This improvement is particularly beneficial in areas with complex flow patterns or in patients with high heart rates, where traditional black-blood techniques might struggle.

Comparative Advantages over Two-dimensional Imaging

The transition from 2D to 3D black-blood MR imaging brings several notable advantages. First, the volumetric acquisition of 3D MR imaging allows for complete coverage of the target vessel segment in a single scan, eliminating the slice-by-slice approach of 2D imaging. This comprehensive coverage reduces the risk of missing small or eccentric plaques and provides a more accurate assessment of plaque burden and distribution.

Another advantage is the reduction in scan time and improved patient comfort. Although 3D sequences can be inherently longer, the need for fewer repeat scans due to comprehensive coverage and the use of accelerated imaging techniques can result in a shorter overall examination time.

The higher spatial resolution of 3D black-blood MR imaging provides more detailed visualization of plaque morphology and composition. This level of detail is crucial for identifying high-risk plaque features, such as thin fibrous caps or necrotic cores, which are predictors of plaque rupture and subsequent cardiovascular events.

Furthermore, 3D imaging facilitates multiplanar reconstruction, allowing clinicians to view the vessel wall and plaques from various angles and planes. This capability is invaluable in presurgical planning and in situations where complex anatomic relationships need to be delineated.

Clinical Applications and Case Studies

Clinically, 3D black-blood MR imaging has found applications in various aspects of cardiovascular care.[21] It is particularly useful in the comprehensive assessment of carotid artery disease, where it can aid in stroke risk stratification. In cases where 2D imaging provides ambiguous results, 3D imaging can offer clarity by providing detailed views of the plaque and its relationship to the surrounding structures.

A notable case study involves the use of 3D black-blood MR imaging in evaluating patients with suspected carotid artery stenosis. The technique provided detailed images of the plaque composition and morphology, aiding in the decision-making process for surgical intervention. In this case, the 3D images revealed a significant soft plaque with a high risk of rupture, which was not clearly evident in the 2D images, leading to a timely and life-saving carotid endarterectomy.[22,23]

In another instance, 3D black-blood MR imaging was employed to monitor plaque progression in a patient undergoing statin therapy. The technique provided clear evidence of plaque regression over time, demonstrating the therapeutic efficacy and guiding further management.[24]

In conclusion, 3D black-blood MR imaging has emerged as a powerful tool in the arsenal of vascular imaging. Its ability to provide detailed, high-resolution images of the entire vessel wall and plaque, combined with a patient-friendly approach, positions it as a superior alternative to the traditional 2D imaging. As this technology continues to evolve, its application in clinical practice is expected to expand, offering new insights into the diagnosis, management, and understanding of vascular diseases.

TWO-DIMENSIONAL VERSUS THREE-DIMENSIONAL IMAGING IN VASCULAR MR IMAGING
Comparative Analysis of 2D and 3D Techniques

The choice between 2D and 3D black-blood MR imaging techniques in vascular imaging is influenced by their distinct capabilities and limitations. Two-dimensional MR imaging, with its high spatial resolution and excellent blood signal suppression, has long been the standard in vessel wall imaging. It excels in providing detailed images of the vessel wall and plaque composition, essential for diagnosing various vascular conditions. However, 2D MR imaging is limited by its slice-by-slice acquisition method, which can be time-consuming and prone to misregistration errors due to patient's movements or blood flow.

On the other hand, 3D MR imaging offers volumetric data acquisition, capturing the entire length of the vessel in a single scan. This comprehensive coverage reduces the risk of missing lesions and provides a more complete picture of the vessel's condition. The ability to reconstruct images in multiple planes further enhances the utility of 3D MR imaging. However, the spatial resolution of 3D MR imaging, while improving, is generally considered lower than that of 2D MR imaging.[25] Additionally, 3D scans can be more susceptible to motion artifacts, particularly in areas near the heart or lungs.

Clinical Decision-Making Based on Imaging Choice

The decision to use 2D or 3D MR imaging depends on several factors, including the clinical scenario,

the specific vessel being imaged, and the patient's condition. For instance, 2D MR imaging might be preferred in cases where high-resolution images are required to assess small, detailed structures or when evaluating areas not significantly affected by motion. This makes 2D MR imaging particularly suitable for imaging the carotid arteries, where detailed plaque characterization is crucial.[26]

In contrast, 3D MR imaging is often the technique of choice for imaging longer segments of vessels, such as the aorta or peripheral arteries, where comprehensive coverage is essential.[27] Its ability to provide a complete view of the vessel in a single scan makes it ideal for evaluating widespread vascular diseases or for presurgical planning.

The choice of technique is also influenced by patient-specific factors. For example, in patients who may have difficulty remaining still for extended periods, the shorter scan time of 3D MR imaging could be advantageous.

Future Perspectives in 2D and 3D MR Imaging Technologies

Looking ahead, the development of both 2D and 3D MR imaging technologies continues to evolve rapidly. Advances in MR imaging hardware and software, such as higher field strengths and more sophisticated pulse sequences, are expected to further enhance the spatial resolution of 3D MR imaging while reducing scan times. This will narrow the gap between the 2 techniques in terms of image quality and practicality.

Simultaneously, efforts are underway to mitigate the limitations of 2D MR imaging, particularly concerning scan time and coverage. Techniques such as accelerated imaging and motion correction algorithms are being developed to make 2D MR imaging more efficient and less prone to artifacts.

In the future, we may see a more tailored approach to imaging, where the choice between 2D MR imaging and 3D MR imaging is based not only on the anatomic region or disease process but also on a detailed analysis of each patient's specific needs and circumstances. The integration of artificial intelligence and machine learning in image processing could further enhance the diagnostic capabilities of both techniques, leading to more personalized and effective patient care.[28]

In conclusion, both 2D and 3D MR imaging techniques have their respective strengths and weaknesses, and the choice between them should be based on the specific clinical context and patient factors. As MR imaging technology advances, it is likely that both 2D and 3D techniques will continue to play vital roles in vascular imaging, with their capabilities being further refined and expanded.

PLAQUE COMPOSITION ANALYSIS
Importance of Determining Plaque Composition

Determining the composition of atherosclerotic plaque is crucial in assessing the risk of cardiovascular events such as heart attacks and strokes. Plaques composed of different materials exhibit varied levels of stability; for instance, plaques with a large lipid core and thin fibrous cap are more prone to rupture, leading to acute events.[29,30] Conversely, plaques rich in fibrous tissue tend to be more stable.[31,32] Understanding plaque composition allows clinicians to stratify patients' risk more accurately, tailor treatment strategies, and monitor the progression or regression of the disease under therapeutic interventions.[33,34]

Role of T1 and T2 Relaxometry in Plaque Characterization

MR imaging relaxometry, involving T1 and T2 relaxation time measurements, is a powerful tool in the characterization of atherosclerotic plaque composition. T1 and T2 relaxometry provides information about the molecular environment within tissues based on how quickly protons in different tissue components return to their equilibrium state after being disturbed by the MR imaging radiofrequency pulse.

T1 relaxometry is particularly useful in identifying lipid-rich areas within plaques. Lipids have a shorter T1 relaxation time compared to other tissue components, which makes them appear brighter in T1-weighted images.[35] This property is exploited to detect lipid cores within atherosclerotic plaques, an essential feature of high-risk, unstable plaques.[36] Additionally, T1-weighted imaging is beneficial in detecting intraplaque hemorrhage, another marker of plaque vulnerability.[37,38]

T2 relaxometry, on the other hand, is effective in identifying fibrous and calcified components of the plaque. Fibrous tissues have longer T2 relaxation times and appear darker on T2-weighted images, whereas calcifications, having very short T2 relaxation times, appear as signal voids.[39–42] The ability to distinguish these components is vital in assessing plaque stability and evaluating the effectiveness of certain treatments, like statins, which can change the composition of plaques over time.[43]

Diffusion-weighted Imaging in Plaque Assessment

DWI is another MR imaging technique that enhances plaque characterization. DWI assesses the diffusion of water molecules within tissues, which varies depending on the tissue's cellular structure and density.[44] In the context of plaque analysis, DWI can provide information about the cellular composition of the plaque, particularly the presence of a high-density macrophage population, which is often associated with inflammation and plaque instability.[45]

High signal intensity on DWI within a plaque suggests increased cellular density and reduced diffusion, often indicative of active inflammation. This information can be pivotal in identifying vulnerable plaques that are at an increased risk of rupture. Moreover, DWI can be used in conjunction with other MR imaging techniques, like T1 and T2 relaxometry, to provide a comprehensive picture of plaque composition and stability.[46]

In conclusion, the analysis of plaque composition using MR imaging relaxometry and DWI plays a critical role in the management of atherosclerotic disease. These techniques offer a noninvasive means to assess plaque characteristics, providing valuable insights into the risk of cardiovascular events and the effectiveness of therapeutic interventions. As MR imaging technology continues to advance, the precision and utility of these imaging techniques in plaque characterization are expected to enhance, leading to better patient outcomes in the management of cardiovascular diseases.

PERMEABILITY QUANTIFICATION WITH DCE-MR IMAGING
Principles of DCE-MR imaging

DCE-MR imaging is an advanced imaging technique used to evaluate the permeability of biological tissues, particularly in the context of vascular diseases.[47,48] The core principle of DCE-MR imaging involves the intravenous administration of a contrast agent, typically gadolinium-based, and the subsequent imaging of its passage through the tissue of interest.

As the contrast agent circulates, it temporarily alters the magnetic properties of blood and tissue, which can be detected by MR imaging. By acquiring rapid, sequential images of the area of interest, DCE-MR imaging captures the dynamics of the contrast agent's distribution and washout. These data are then analyzed to derive quantitative measures of tissue perfusion and permeability.[49] The rate and extent to which the contrast agent accumulates within the tissue—and how quickly it washes out—provide valuable information about the microvascular structure and permeability of the tissue.

Clinical Significance of Permeability Measurement

In the assessment of atherosclerotic plaque, the measurement of vessel wall permeability through

DCE-MR imaging has significant clinical implications. High permeability is often indicative of a compromised endothelial barrier and increased neovascularization within the plaque, both of which are markers of plaque vulnerability and inflammation. Vulnerable plaques are prone to rupture, leading to acute cardiovascular events such as myocardial infarctions or strokes.

By quantifying permeability, DCE-MR imaging helps in identifying high-risk plaques, thus aiding in the risk stratification of patients.[49,50] This information can be pivotal in making clinical decisions, such as the intensity of medical therapy or the need for surgical interventions. Furthermore, DCE-MR imaging is instrumental in research settings, where it is used to study the pathophysiology of atherosclerosis and to evaluate the efficacy of antiatherosclerotic drugs.

Challenges and Advancements in DCE-MR imaging Techniques

While DCE-MR imaging is a powerful tool for assessing vascular permeability, it presents several challenges. One of the primary challenges is the need for precise timing and rapid imaging sequences to accurately capture the dynamics of contrast agent distribution. This requirement often necessitates the use of high-end MR imaging scanners and sophisticated imaging protocols, which may not be readily available in all clinical settings.

Another challenge is the interpretation of DCE-MR imaging data, which can be complex and requires sophisticated modeling to extract meaningful permeability metrics.[51] The accuracy of these models can be influenced by various factors, including the type of contrast agent used, the patient's hemodynamic status, and the specific imaging parameters employed.

Despite these challenges, significant advancements have been made in DCE-MR imaging techniques. Improved imaging sequences and faster MR imaging scanners have made it possible to acquire higher resolution images more quickly, enhancing the accuracy of permeability measurements. Additionally, the development of more sophisticated contrast agents and data analysis algorithms has improved the sensitivity and specificity of DCE-MR imaging in detecting subtle changes in tissue permeability.

Emerging techniques, such as the use of artificial intelligence and machine learning in image analysis, are expected to further streamline the interpretation of DCE-MR imaging data and enhance its clinical applicability. Ongoing research into novel contrast agents that specifically target certain components

of the plaque could also provide more detailed insights into plaque pathology.[52]

In conclusion, DCE-MR imaging is a valuable tool in the assessment of vascular permeability, offering critical insights into plaque vulnerability and the risk of cardiovascular events. Despite its challenges, ongoing technological and methodological advancements continue to expand its capabilities, solidifying its role in the diagnosis and management of vascular diseases.

ALTERNATIVE TECHNIQUES FOR MEASURING PERMEABILITY
Overview of Alternative Imaging Modalities

While DCE-MR imaging is a prominent method for assessing vascular permeability, several other imaging modalities offer alternative approaches. These include PET, CT, ultrasound imaging with contrast agents, and optical coherence tomography (OCT).

PET: PET, often combined with CT (PET/CT), utilizes radioactive tracers to assess metabolic activity and blood flow, providing insights into tissue permeability. It is particularly useful in oncology for tumor imaging but is increasingly being explored for vascular imaging.[53]

CT: CT, especially with the use of contrast agents, can provide information about blood flow and vessel wall characteristics. CT angiography is widely used for assessing large vessel diseases but has limitations in evaluating microvascular permeability.

Ultrasound imaging with contrast agents: This technique involves the use of microbubble contrast agents that enhance ultrasound signals. It is useful for assessing blood flow and can provide some information about permeability, particularly in superficial vessels.

OCT: OCT is a noninvasive imaging technique that provides high-resolution images of small vessels. It is primarily used in ophthalmology but has potential applications in assessing superficial vascular structures.

Comparative Analysis with DCE-MR imaging

Sensitivity and resolution: DCE-MR imaging provides high-resolution images and is highly sensitive in detecting changes in tissue permeability. PET and OCT also offer high sensitivity but are limited in spatial resolution (PET) and depth of penetration (OCT). CT and ultrasound are less sensitive than DCE-MR imaging for microvascular changes but are useful in larger vessels.

Specificity: DCE-MR imaging offers detailed tissue characterization, which is advantageous in distinguishing between different types of vascular pathologies. PET provides metabolic information, which can be beneficial in certain clinical scenarios. CT and ultrasound are less specific for tissue characterization compared to DCE-MR imaging and PET.

Accessibility and safety: CT and ultrasound are more widely available and have shorter scan times compared to DCE-MR imaging. However, CT involves ionizing radiation, and some ultrasound contrast agents may have limitations in patients with specific allergies or cardiac conditions. DCE-MR imaging and PET are more specialized and less accessible but offer radiation-free imaging (DCE-MR imaging) and unique metabolic insights (PET).

Cost and practicality: DCE-MR imaging and PET are generally more expensive and less widely available than CT and ultrasound. OCT is also limited in its applicability to certain vascular beds due to its depth limitation.

Clinical Implications of Different Techniques

The choice of imaging modality for assessing vascular permeability depends on the clinical context, the specific vascular territory being evaluated, patient factors, and resource availability. DCE-MR imaging is preferred for detailed tissue characterization and when high-resolution images of microvascular structures are required. PET/CT may be advantageous in oncological applications or when metabolic information is crucial. CT and ultrasound are more suitable for rapid, large-scale screening and in situations where DCE-MR imaging is not available or feasible.

In conclusion, while DCE-MR imaging remains a cornerstone in permeability assessment, each of alternative imaging techniques brings unique strengths and limitations. The choice of modality should be guided by the specific clinical needs, availability of resources, and the overall goals of the vascular assessment. As imaging technology advances, the integration of multiple modalities may offer complementary insights, leading to more comprehensive vascular evaluations.

FLOW-DERIVED BIOMECHANICAL WALL PARAMETERS
Importance of Wall Shear Stress and Arterial Stiffness

The biomechanical properties of blood vessels, such as wall shear stress (WSS) and arterial stiffness, play critical roles in vascular health and disease. WSS, the tangential force exerted by blood flow on the vessel wall, influences endothelial cell function, plaque formation, and progression. Abnormal WSS, whether too high or too low, can promote atherosclerosis and is a crucial factor in plaque vulnerability.[54]

Arterial stiffness, reflecting the rigidity of vessel walls, is a key marker of cardiovascular risk and aging. Increased arterial stiffness is associated with various pathologies, including hypertension, stroke, and myocardial infarction.[55] It affects how blood pressure waves propagate through the vasculature, influencing organ perfusion and cardiac workload.

MR Imaging Techniques in Measuring Biomechanical Parameters

Phase-contrast MR (PC-MR) imaging: This technique is extensively used to measure blood flow velocity, from which WSS can be derived. PC-MR imaging captures the movement of blood through the vascular system, allowing for the calculation of velocity gradients near the vessel walls.[56] These gradients are used to estimate WSS, providing insights into the hemodynamic forces acting on the endothelium.[57]

Cine MR imaging: Cine MR imaging, particularly when combined with PC-MR imaging, helps in assessing arterial stiffness. By imaging the vessel wall movement throughout the cardiac cycle, cine MR imaging can determine parameters like pulse wave velocity (PWV)—a direct measure of arterial stiffness. PWV is calculated by measuring the speed of the blood pressure wave between 2 points in the vascular system.

Black-blood MR imaging with elastography: This technique provides direct measurement of vessel wall stiffness. Black-blood MR imaging suppresses the blood signal, focusing on the vessel wall, while elastography measures the wall's mechanical properties, such as strain and stiffness, in response to pulsatile pressure.

Clinical Relevance and Research Applications

The clinical relevance of measuring WSS and arterial stiffness is profound. Abnormal WSS is a predictor of regions prone to atherosclerotic plaque development and can guide interventions to modify risk factors or direct therapeutic strategies.[58] For instance, in patients with coronary artery disease, regions of low WSS might be targeted for more aggressive medical therapy or monitored more closely.

Arterial stiffness measurements are crucial in managing hypertension and predicting cardiovascular events.[59] Stiffness parameters can guide the choice of antihypertensive medications, as some drugs may be more effective in reducing stiffness than others. Moreover, stiffness measurements are useful in evaluating the effectiveness of interventions aimed at improving vascular health.

In research, these measurements are invaluable in understanding the pathophysiology of vascular diseases. Studies on WSS can shed light on the mechanisms of plaque initiation and progression, while research on arterial stiffness contributes to our understanding of aging and its impact on the cardiovascular system.

Recent advancements in MR imaging technology, including higher field strengths and more sophisticated analysis algorithms, have improved the accuracy and utility of these measurements. Moreover, the development of noninvasive, radiation-free techniques for assessing WSS and arterial stiffness makes MR imaging an attractive modality for both clinical and research applications.

In conclusion, the assessment of flow-derived biomechanical wall parameters using MR imaging techniques is vital in understanding and managing vascular diseases. These measurements provide crucial insights into the forces shaping vascular health and the risk of cardiovascular events, influencing both clinical decision-making and research directions in vascular medicine. As MR imaging technology continues to evolve, its application in evaluating biomechanical parameters is expected to grow, offering new opportunities for enhancing cardiovascular health.

SUMMARY
Summary of Key Findings

This comprehensive review underscores the integral role of MR imaging in the characterization of vessel walls, a pivotal aspect of vascular medicine. The advancements in MR imaging technology, particularly in the domains of black-blood MR imaging, both 2D and 3D, and DCE-MR imaging, have significantly enhanced our ability to visualize and quantify vascular pathologies noninvasively.

Two-dimensional black-blood MR imaging, with its high spatial resolution, remains a cornerstone in detailed plaque characterization, offering insights into plaque stability and risk. The advent of 3D black-blood MR imaging, while slightly compromising on resolution, provides volumetric data acquisition, enabling comprehensive vessel wall assessment in a single scan. DCE-MR imaging emerges as a sophisticated tool for evaluating vascular permeability, offering crucial insights into plaque vulnerability and inflammation.

Furthermore, the assessment of biomechanical properties like WSS and arterial stiffness through phase-contrast and cine MR imaging techniques has opened new avenues in understanding the pathophysiology of vascular diseases and guiding therapeutic interventions. These advancements reflect MR imaging's unparalleled ability to provide detailed anatomic, compositional, and functional information about the vessel wall, making it an invaluable modality in the diagnosis and management of vascular diseases.

Future Directions in MR Imaging-based Vessel Wall Characterization

Looking ahead, the future of MR imaging-based vessel wall characterization is poised for significant advancements. The integration of higher field strengths, advanced imaging sequences, and artificial intelligence for image analysis promises to further enhance the resolution, speed, and accuracy of MR imaging. This progress will likely narrow the gaps in current imaging capabilities, such as the resolution limitations of 3D imaging or the complexity of DCE-MR imaging interpretation.

Emerging technologies, such as hybrid imaging systems combining MR imaging with other modalities like PET, may provide complementary insights into vascular pathologies. Additionally, the development of novel contrast agents and molecular imaging techniques could allow for more targeted imaging of specific plaque components or biological processes.[60]

Final Thoughts on the Impact of MR Imaging in Vascular Medicine

MR imaging's impact on vascular medicine cannot be overstated. It has revolutionized our approach to diagnosing and managing vascular diseases, moving beyond mere luminal assessment to a comprehensive evaluation of vessel wall health. The ability to noninvasively characterize vessel walls in such detail has not only enhanced clinical care but has also propelled research in vascular pathophysiology.

As we advance, MR imaging is expected to remain at the forefront of vascular imaging, continually evolving and adapting to meet the challenges of this dynamic field. Its ongoing development will undoubtedly contribute to improved patient outcomes, deeper understanding of vascular diseases, and the advancement of personalized medicine in vascular health care.

CLINICS CARE POINTS

- Black-blood MR imaging is valuable in identifying various plaque components such as the fibrous cap, lipid core, and calcifications.
- Diffusion-weighted imaging can provide information about the cellular composition of the plaque which is often associated with inflammation and plaque instability.

- Biomechanical properties such as wall shear stress and arterial stiffness can be measured with MR imaging techniques and play a role in plaque formation and progression.

DISCLOSURE

I have no relationship with a commercial company that has a direct financial interest in the subject matter or materials discussed in this article or with a company making a competing product.

REFERENCES

1. Harteveld AA, Denswil NP, Siero JC, et al. Quantitative Intracranial Atherosclerotic Plaque Characterization at 7T MRI: An Ex Vivo Study with Histologic Validation. AJNR Am J Neuroradiol 2016;37:802–10.
2. Singh N, Moody AR, Roifman I, et al. Advanced MRI for carotid plaque imaging. Int J Cardiovasc Imag 2016;32:83–9.
3. Bos D, Arshi B, van den Bouwhuijsen QJA, et al. Atherosclerotic Carotid Plaque Composition and Incident Stroke and Coronary Events. J Am Coll Cardiol 2021;77:1426–35.
4. Dweck MR, Puntman V, Vesey AT, et al. MR Imaging of Coronary Arteries and Plaques. JACC Cardiovasc Imaging 2016;9:306–16.
5. He Y, Da QY, An J, et al. Coronary artery plaque imaging: Comparison of black-blood MRI and 64-multidetector computed tomography. Chronic Dis Transl Med 2016;2:159–65.
6. Edelman RR, Chien D, Kim D. Fast selective black blood MR imaging. Radiology 1991;181:655–60.
7. Itskovich VV, Mani V, Mizsei G, et al. Parallel and nonparallel simultaneous multislice black-blood double inversion recovery techniques for vessel wall imaging. J Magn Reson Imag 2004;19:459–67.
8. Yarnykh VL, Yuan C. T1-insensitive flow suppression using quadruple inversion-recovery. Magn Reson Med 2002;48:899–905.
9. Takano K, Yamashita S, Takemoto K, et al. Characterization of carotid atherosclerosis with black-blood carotid plaque imaging using variable flip-angle 3D turbo spin-echo: comparison with 2D turbo spin-echo sequences. Eur J Radiol 2012;81:e304–9.
10. Murata K, Murata N, Chu B, et al. Characterization of Carotid Atherosclerotic Plaques Using 3-Dimensional MERGE Magnetic Resonance Imaging and Correlation With Stroke Risk Factors. Stroke 2020;51:475–80.
11. Shu JE, Ying ML, Chen XR, et al. Prognostic value of high-resolution magnetic resonance imaging in evaluating carotid atherosclerotic plaque in patients with ischemic stroke. Medicine (Baltim) 2017;96:e8515.
12. Zhao XQ, Sun J, Hippe DS, et al. Magnetic Resonance Imaging of Intraplaque Hemorrhage and Plaque Lipid Content With Continued Lipid-Lowering Therapy: Results of a Magnetic Resonance Imaging Substudy in AIM-HIGH. Circ Cardiovasc Imaging 2022;15:e014229.
13. Lin K, Lloyd-Jones DM, Bi X, et al. Effects of respiratory motion on coronary wall MR imaging: a quantitative study of older adults. Int J Cardiovasc Imag 2013;29:1069–76.
14. Ning Z, Chen S, Sun H, et al. Evaluating renal arterial wall by non-enhanced 2D and 3D free-breathing black-blood techniques: Initial experience. Magn Reson Imaging 2021;79:5–12.
15. Fan Z, Zhang Z, Chung YC, et al. Carotid arterial wall MRI at 3T using 3D variable-flip-angle turbo spin-echo (TSE) with flow-sensitive dephasing (FSD). J Magn Reson Imag 2010;31:645–54.
16. Eikendal AL, Blomberg BA, Haaring C, et al. 3D black blood VISTA vessel wall cardiovascular magnetic resonance of the thoracic aorta wall in young, healthy adults: reproducibility and implications for efficacy trial sample sizes: a cross-sectional study. J Cardiovasc Magn Reson 2016;18:20.
17. van der Kolk AG, Hendrikse J, Brundel M, et al. Multi-sequence whole-brain intracranial vessel wall imaging at 7.0 tesla. Eur Radiol 2013;23:2996–3004.
18. Li L, Chai JT, Biasiolli L, et al. Black-blood multicontrast imaging of carotid arteries with DANTE-prepared 2D and 3D MR imaging. Radiology 2014;273:560–9.
19. Yoneyama M, Nakamura M, Takahara T, et al. Improvement of T1 contrast in whole-brain black-blood imaging using motion-sensitized driven-equilibrium prepared 3D turbo spin echo (3D MSDE-TSE). Magn Reson Med Sci 2014;13:61–5.
20. Jun C, Shuhua L, Xue Z, et al. Application of motion-sensitized driven equilibrium based black blood 3D TSE sequence in the detection of brain metastases. Magn Reson Imaging 2022;93:145–8.
21. Koktzoglou I, Li D. Diffusion-prepared segmented steady-state free precession: Application to 3D black-blood cardiovascular magnetic resonance of the thoracic aorta and carotid artery walls. J Cardiovasc Magn Reson 2007;9:33–42.
22. Oki S, Ito M, Gekka M, et al. Carotid Endarterectomy for a Case with an Extremely Twisted Internal Carotid Artery. JMA J 2023;6:548–51.
23. Kuroda H, Nakai Y, Miyake S, et al. Feasibility of Preoperative Magnetic Resonance Angiography/Black-Blood Magnetic Resonance Imaging/Computed Tomography Fusion Imaging Without Contrast Agent for Carotid Endarterectomy. World Neurosurg 2022;167:e1219–24.
24. Zhou P, Wang Y, Sun J, et al. Assessment of Therapeutic Response to Statin Therapy in Patients With Intracranial or Extracranial Carotid Atherosclerosis by

Vessel Wall MRI: A Systematic Review and Updated Meta-Analysis. Front Cardiovasc Med 2021;8:742935.

25. Eiden S, Beck C, Venhoff N, et al. High-resolution contrast-enhanced vessel wall imaging in patients with suspected cerebral vasculitis: Prospective comparison of whole-brain 3D T1 SPACE versus 2D T1 black blood MRI at 3 Tesla. PLoS One 2019; 14:e0213514.

26. Balu N, Chu B, Hatsukami TS, et al. Comparison between 2D and 3D high-resolution black-blood techniques for carotid artery wall imaging in clinically significant atherosclerosis. J Magn Reson Imag 2008;27:918–24.

27. Mooiweer R, Sbrizzi A, El Aidi H, et al. Fast 3D isotropic imaging of the aortic vessel wall by application of 2D spatially selective excitation and a new way of inversion recovery for black blood imaging. Magn Reson Med 2016;75:547–55.

28. Cao X, Zeng Y, Wang J, et al. Differentiation of Cerebral Dissecting Aneurysm from Hemorrhagic Saccular Aneurysm by Machine-Learning Based on Vessel Wall MRI: A Multicenter Study. J Clin Med 2022;11.

29. Cai JM, Hatsukami TS, Ferguson MS, et al. Classification of human carotid atherosclerotic lesions with in vivo multicontrast magnetic resonance imaging. Circulation 2002;106:1368–73.

30. Dilba K, van Dam-Nolen DHK, van Dijk AC, et al. Plaque Composition as a Predictor of Plaque Ulceration in Carotid Artery Atherosclerosis: The Plaque At RISK Study. AJNR Am J Neuroradiol 2021;42: 144–51.

31. Catalano O, Bendotti G, Mori A, et al. Evolving determinants of carotid atherosclerosis vulnerability in asymptomatic patients from the MAGNETIC observational study. Sci Rep 2021;11:2327.

32. Chai JT, Biasiolli L, Li L, et al. Quantification of Lipid-Rich Core in Carotid Atherosclerosis Using Magnetic Resonance T(2) Mapping: Relation to Clinical Presentation. JACC Cardiovasc Imaging 2017;10: 747–56.

33. Chen H, Ricks J, Rosenfeld M, et al. Progression of experimental lesions of atherosclerosis: assessment by kinetic modeling of black-blood dynamic contrast-enhanced MRI. Magn Reson Med 2013; 69:1712–20.

34. Corti R, Fuster V, Fayad ZA, et al. Lipid lowering by simvastatin induces regression of human atherosclerotic lesions: two years' follow-up by high-resolution noninvasive magnetic resonance imaging. Circulation 2002;106:2884–7.

35. Messroghli DR, Radjenovic A, Kozerke S, et al. Modified Look-Locker inversion recovery (MOLLI) for high-resolution T1 mapping of the heart. Magn Reson Med 2004;52:141–6.

36. Coolen BF, Poot DH, Liem MI, et al. Three-dimensional quantitative T1 and T2 mapping of the carotid artery: Sequence design and in vivo feasibility. Magn Reson Med 2016;75:1008–17.

37. Koning W, de Rotte AA, Bluemink JJ, et al. MRI of the carotid artery at 7 Tesla: quantitative comparison with 3 Tesla. J Magn Reson Imag 2015;41:773–80.

38. Wang J, Bornert P, Zhao H, et al. Simultaneous non-contrast angiography and intraplaque hemorrhage (SNAP) imaging for carotid atherosclerotic disease evaluation. Magn Reson Med 2013;69:337–45.

39. Chu B, Kampschulte A, Ferguson MS, et al. Hemorrhage in the atherosclerotic carotid plaque: a high-resolution MRI study. Stroke 2004;35:1079–84.

40. Toussaint JF, LaMuraglia GM, Southern JF, et al. Magnetic resonance images lipid, fibrous, calcified, hemorrhagic, and thrombotic components of human atherosclerosis in vivo. Circulation 1996; 94:932–8.

41. Biasiolli L, Lindsay AC, Chai JT, et al. In-vivo quantitative T2 mapping of carotid arteries in atherosclerotic patients: segmentation and T2 measurement of plaque components. J Cardiovasc Magn Reson 2013;15:69.

42. Raman SV, Winner MW 3rd, Tran T, et al. In vivo atherosclerotic plaque characterization using magnetic susceptibility distinguishes symptom-producing plaques. JACC Cardiovasc Imaging 2008;1:49–57.

43. Tang TY, Howarth SP, Miller SR, et al. The ATHEROMA (Atorvastatin Therapy: Effects on Reduction of Macrophage Activity) Study. Evaluation using ultrasmall superparamagnetic iron oxide-enhanced magnetic resonance imaging in carotid disease. J Am Coll Cardiol 2009;53:2039–50.

44. Toussaint JF, Southern JF, Fuster V, et al. Water diffusion properties of human atherosclerosis and thrombosis measured by pulse field gradient nuclear magnetic resonance. Arterioscler Thromb Vasc Biol 1997;17:542–6.

45. Qiao Y, Ronen I, Viereck J, et al. Identification of atherosclerotic lipid deposits by diffusion-weighted imaging. Arterioscler Thromb Vasc Biol 2007;27: 1440–6.

46. Clarke SE, Hammond RR, Mitchell JR, et al. Quantitative assessment of carotid plaque composition using multicontrast MRI and registered histology. Magn Reson Med 2003;50:1199–208.

47. van Hoof RH, Heeneman S, Wildberger JE, et al. Dynamic Contrast-Enhanced MRI to Study Atherosclerotic Plaque Microvasculature. Curr Atheroscler Rep 2016;18:33.

48. Ruparelia N, Chai JT, Fisher EA, et al. Inflammatory processes in cardiovascular disease: a route to targeted therapies. Nat Rev Cardiol 2017;14:133–44.

49. Kerwin WS, O'Brien KD, Ferguson MS, et al. Inflammation in carotid atherosclerotic plaque: a dynamic contrast-enhanced MR imaging study. Radiology 2006;241:459–68.

50. Gaens ME, Backes WH, Rozel S, et al. Dynamic contrast-enhanced MR imaging of carotid atherosclerotic plaque: model selection, reproducibility, and validation. Radiology 2013;266:271–9.

51. van Hoof RHM, Voo SA, Sluimer JC, et al. Vessel wall and adventitial DCE-MRI parameters demonstrate similar correlations with carotid plaque microvasculature on histology. J Magn Reson Imag 2017;46:1053–9.

52. Calcagno C, Lairez O, Hawkins J, et al. Combined PET/DCE-MRI in a Rabbit Model of Atherosclerosis: Integrated Quantification of Plaque Inflammation, Permeability, and Burden During Treatment With a Leukotriene A4 Hydrolase Inhibitor. JACC Cardiovasc Imaging 2018;11:291–301.

53. Senders ML, Hernot S, Carlucci G, et al. Nanobody-Facilitated Multiparametric PET/MRI Phenotyping of Atherosclerosis. JACC Cardiovasc Imaging 2019;12:2015–26.

54. Malek AM, Alper SL, Izumo S. Hemodynamic shear stress and its role in atherosclerosis. JAMA 1999;282:2035–42.

55. Kroner ES, Lamb HJ, Siebelink HM, et al. Pulse wave velocity and flow in the carotid artery versus the aortic arch: effects of aging. J Magn Reson Imag 2014;40:287–93.

56. Oshinski JN, Ku DN, Mukundan S Jr, et al. Determination of wall shear stress in the aorta with the use of MR phase velocity mapping. J Magn Reson Imag 1995;5:640–7.

57. Oyre S, Ringgaard S, Kozerke S, et al. Quantitation of circumferential subpixel vessel wall position and wall shear stress by multiple sectored three-dimensional paraboloid modeling of velocity encoded cine MR. Magn Reson Med 1998;40:645–55.

58. Markl M, Wegent F, Zech T, et al. In vivo wall shear stress distribution in the carotid artery: effect of bifurcation geometry, internal carotid artery stenosis, and recanalization therapy. Circ Cardiovasc Imaging 2010;3:647–55.

59. van Popele NMG DE, Bots ML, Asmar R, et al. Association between arterial stiffness and atherosclerosis: the Rotterdam Study. Stroke 2001;32:454–60.

60. Duivenvoorden R, Tang J, Cormode DP, et al. A statin-loaded reconstituted high-density lipoprotein nanoparticle inhibits atherosclerotic plaque inflammation. Nat Commun 2014;5:3065.

Printed and bound by CPI Group (UK) Ltd, Croydon, CR0 4YY

03/10/2024

01040367-0005